**Nour Elhouda Souissi**
**Mohamed Hedi Ben Cheikh**

**Container-content interactions**

Nour Elhouda Souissi
Mohamed Hedi Ben Cheikh

# Container-content interactions

## Theoretical and practical aspects

ScienciaScripts

Cover image: www.ingimage.com

This book is a translation from the original published under ISBN 978-3-639-52448-2.

Publisher:
Sciencia Scripts
is a trademark of
Dodo Books Indian Ocean Ltd. and OmniScriptum S.R.L publishing group

120 High Road, East Finchley, London, N2 9ED, United Kingdom
Str. Armeneasca 28/1, office 1, Chisinau MD-2012, Republic of Moldova, Europe
Managing Directors: Ieva Konstantinova, Victoria Ursu
info@omniscriptum.com

Printed at: see last page
**ISBN: 978-620-8-53710-4**

# CONTENTS

# INTRODUCTION

Before they can be marketed, medicines must meet strict quality, efficacy and safety requirements. They must demonstrate their stability and ability to be stored properly from manufacture to use.

However, various internal and external factors could compromise their quality, including environmental factors (temperature, light, humidity, oxygen), interactions between the various constituents (active substances and excipients) and incompatibilities between their galenic forms and packaging **[1]**.

Incompatibilities between drugs and their packaging are known as "container-content interactions" (CCI). The first documented case dates back to the early $^{20th}$ century, when a decrease in the levels of two bacteriostatic products (phenol and cresol) contained in glass bottles fitted with rubber stoppers was described **[2]**. Investigations revealed that these products had been absorbed by the stoppers.

With the emergence of plastic medical packaging and devices (syringes, bags, infusion lines, etc.), the number of CCI-related incidents has continued to grow **[3]**. Although these new products have solved serious problems often encountered with their glass counterparts, such as the risk of microbial contamination or the risk of gas embolism associated with glass containers, plastic devices have also led to the emergence of CCI phenomena. Indeed, cases of loss of active ingredients through sorption on plastic tubing and bags, and release of toxic substances into drugs and blood derivatives from medical packaging and devices, have been reported in many contexts.

Aware of these emerging problems, the scientific community and the relevant authorities have carried out numerous investigations to study CCIs, explain the phenomena involved and the factors favoring their occurrence, assess the toxicity of the substances released and set up analytical methods for their detection and control **[4]**.

In this work, we planned to carry out a literature review on ICCs in order to describe the phenomena involved and their impact on product quality and human health safety, while specifying methodical approaches for their analysis and control. By reporting actual published cases, the main objective was to raise awareness among healthcare professionals of the risks incurred by patients when using a pharmaceutical product incompatible with its container.

# 1. PACKAGING FOR PHARMACEUTICAL USE

Pharmaceutical packaging comes in a wide variety of shapes, forms and sizes. This is due to the variety of routes of administration (oral, parenteral, ophthalmic, cutaneous, etc.) and pharmaceutical forms (solid, liquid and semi-solid). Commonly used packaging types include :

- Bottles for liquid forms;
- Blisters for tablets and capsules;
- Sachets for powders and granules;
- Tubes for semi-solid shapes.

On the other hand, these packages are classified into three distinct groups **[5]** :

- **Primary packaging:** contains medicines and is in direct contact with them;
- **Secondary packaging:** contains primary packaging and auxiliary components such as spoons, measuring cups and leaflets;
- **Tertiary packaging:** contains several units of medicines packaged in their primary and secondary packaging. They protect medicines during transport, distribution and storage.

Pharmaceutical packaging is made from a wide range of materials (glass, plastics, elastomers, metals, etc.). Each material is distinguished by physico-chemical properties which subsequently determine its use.

## 1.1. The glass

Glass is widely used in the pharmaceutical industry. It is used to package a wide range of galenic forms (oral solutions and suspensions, syrups, powders and injectable solutions, etc.) and comes in the form of vials, ampoules, cartridges and pre-filled syringes.

Glass is an inorganic material **[6]**. It is obtained from a mixture of substances heated to fusion, then cooled to form a non-crystalline (amorphous) solid. The main component of glass is called the "network former". This is often an oxide or a mixture of oxides: silicon oxide ($SiO_2$), boron oxide ($B_2O_3$), phosphorus oxide ($P_2O_5$) or germanium oxide ($GeO_2$). The glasses used in the manufacture of pharmaceutical packaging are based on silicon oxide (silicate glasses).

In its pure state, glass requires excessively high temperatures (above 1700°C) to melt **[7]**. This represents a challenge for industrial production, which has led to the addition of other minerals (lattice modifiers) that lower the melting point of glass, such as sodium oxide and potassium oxide. Other substances, called lattice stabilizers (such as calcium oxide, aluminum oxide), can be added to glass to improve its durability. In addition, metal oxides (iron oxides, titanium oxide and manganese oxide) can be added if a photo-protective effect is required.

Silicate glass, used in the manufacture of packaging for pharmaceutical use, is classified according to its formulation into two main families **[6]** :

- **Calc-sodium glass**: this family is the oldest and most abundant. Calc-sodium glass contains relatively high levels of sodium oxide and calcium oxide (25% of total composition). It may also contain magnesium oxide, potassium oxide and aluminum oxide in lesser proportions;
- **Borosilicate glass** (or neutral glass): this family is distinguished from calcosodium glass by its lower sodium and calcium oxide content, and the addition of boron oxide ($B_2O_3$). The latter gives it greater resistance to thermal shock and hydrolytic attack.

International pharmacopoeias classify glass for pharmaceutical use into three types, according to hydrolytic resistance. According to the European

Pharmacopoeia **[8]**, the hydrolytic resistance of glass is defined as "its resistance to the release of water-soluble mineral substances, under specified conditions of contact between the inner surface of the container or the glass grains and water". Glass for pharmaceutical use is classified as follows **[6,8]**:

- **Type I glass:** has high hydrolytic resistance, due to its chemical composition. Borosilicate glass is a Type I glass.
- **Type II glass:** high hydrolytic resistance thanks to appropriate surface treatment (e.g. application of ammonium sulfate to the inner surface of the glass. This reacts with the alkali and alkaline-earth ions present on the surface to form water-soluble salts, which are then rinsed off.) Type II glass is generally treated calc-sodium glass;
- **Type III glass:** has average hydrolytic resistance and generally corresponds to untreated calc-sodium glass.

Pharmacopoeias also specify the use of each type of glass (**Table I**).

**Table II : Use of glass in pharmaceutical packaging according to type**

| Glass type | Use / Container |
|---|---|
| Type I | Parenteral and non-parenteral preparations. |
| Type II | Parenteral and non-parenteral, acidic or neutral aqueous preparations. |
| Type III | Preparations not intended for parenteral administration ;<br>Non-aqueous preparations for parenteral administration ;<br>Powders for parenteral administration (excluding lyophilized preparations). |

## 1.2. Plastics

Globally, plastics are the most widely used raw materials for pharmaceutical packaging, thanks to their exceptional physico-chemical properties, diversity and cost-effectiveness**[9]**. Plastic packaging components include vials, ampoules, pouches, pre-filled syringes, tubes and closures. Unlike glass, which is relatively heavy, can break easily when handled or stored at low temperatures, and releases alkalis when exposed to aqueous solutions, plastics are lightweight, flexible, unbreakable, can be transparent or opaque, and are easy to shape and seal, giving a wide variety of shapes and sizes and enabling the inclusion of delivery devices.

Plastics belong to a class of materials called polymers, which are organic macromolecules of high molecular weight **[5]**. Each macromolecule is a linear or spatial sequence of small, repeating chemical units (called monomers), linked together by covalent bonds. Monomers can be of the same or different natures. By way of illustration, ethylene can be polymerized on its own to form the homopolymer polyethylene, or it can be reacted with a chemical species distinct from it, such as vinyl acetate, to form the copolymer polyethylene-vinyl acetate. Polymers can be linear, branched or cross-linked, and can be amorphous or semi-crystalline in structure.

Depending on their physical properties, plastic compounds can be divided into two classes: thermoplastics and thermosetting plastics **[5]**. In general, thermoplastics have linear and branched structures, while thermosetting polymers are cross-linked. Thermoplastics commonly used in the pharmaceutical industry include polyolefins, polyethylene, polypropylene, polyethylene terephthalate, polycarbonate and polyvinyl chloride (PVC) **[4]**. Thermosetting plastics include epoxy resins, polyester resins and adhesives.

During polymer production, several chemicals are added to facilitate the monomer polymerization reaction (catalysts, solvents, gas pedals, etc.) **[5]**. These compounds persist in the finished products and are referred to as process residues. Unreacted monomers may also be present. When polymers are processed into packaging components, medical devices or manufacturing equipment, other chemicals are added (these are called additives). These products are added to improve the manufacturing process or the mechanical, physical and chemical properties of polymers. Additives include lubricants, mold release agents, plasticizers, antioxidants, stabilizers, opacifiers, etc. The functions of the main additives are summarized **in Table II**.

**TableII : Main plastic additives and their roles, from[5].**

| Aditif | Role | Examples |
|---|---|---|
| Plasticizers | Improves flow properties; Increases polymer softness and flexibility. | Phthalates |
| Stabilizers | Improves polymer resistance to temperature and light | Calcium and zinc salts |
| Antioxidants | Prevent or retard oxidative degradation of polymers | Crésols |
| Opacifiers | Make polymers opaque | Titanium dioxide |
| Lubricants | Prevent adhesion of plastics to metal parts during manufacturing | Waxes, liquid kerosene |

## 1.3. Elastomers

In pharmaceutical packaging, elastomers are mainly used to manufacture parenteral container closures (vial stoppers, syringe and cartridge seals, syringe tip caps, etc.) **[5]**.

Elastomers are polymers distinguished from plastics by their elasticity, which corresponds to the ability of a given material to return to its initial shape after stretching or deformation **[10]**. Thanks to this property, elastomers are flexible, maintain a seal and reseal after puncturing, hence their use in parenteral container closures.

Elastomers can be natural (extracted from rubber trees) or synthetic (derived from petrochemicals) **[5]**. Elastomers for pharmaceutical use contain the following substances in their formulation:

- **Polymers**: these are the main components of elastomers. An elastomer is composed of a single polymer or a combination of different polymers. Isoprene, isobutylene-isoprene and styrene-butadiene are the polymers most commonly used in pharmaceutical packaging;
- **Vulcanizing** agents (or cross-linking agents): these components impart elasticity to the polymer(s), by establishing chemical bonds between molecules of different polymer chains. There are many types of cross-linking agents, including sulfur, peroxides and amines;
- **Fillers**: these substances impart hardness, reinforcement and strength to elastomers. The most commonly used fillers are inorganic substances such as aluminum or magnesium silicates;
- **Colorants**: these substances impart color to elastomers. Elastomers often come in gray, black or red. The gray color is obtained by mixing titanium oxide (white) with minute quantities of carbon. The red color is imparted by iron oxide;

- **Other components**: plasticizers, antioxidants, antiozonants, etc.

## 1.4. Other materials

Glass, plastics and elastomers are the main materials used in the construction of primary packaging for pharmaceutical use. However, other materials are also used in primary, secondary and tertiary packaging **[5]** :

- **Metals:** aluminum and tinplate (steel foil coated on both sides with tin) are used in drug packaging. Metered-dose aerosols, semi-solid drug tubes and blister packs are examples of packaging systems made entirely or partly of metals. These have a number of advantages: they are strong, can withstand high pressure, and are impermeable to gas and light.
- **Paper:** paper is one of the oldest packaging materials. Among the most common paper packaging components are labels, leaflets and cartons.
- **Laminates:** laminates are obtained by adhering films (layers) of separate materials such as paper, plastics and metals. The aim is to combine the desirable properties of each material into a single CE. Laminates are used to manufacture containers such as sachets, blister packs, tubes and pouches.

# 2. CONTAINER-CONTENT INTERACTIONS

## 2.1. Phenomena involved

Container-content interactions are physico-chemical phenomena that occur when a product (liquid, gas or solid) is brought into contact with a solid material **[11]**. Substances are transferred between the two compartments: from the product (compartment 1) to the material (compartment 2), or vice versa. In addition, substances may migrate from the product through the material to the outside environment, or vice versa. These transfers continue until a state of equilibrium is reached between the two compartments, or until contact between them ceases. The kinetics and amplitude of CCI depend on a number of factors:

- Physicochemical properties of the contents: size, structure, solubility, lipophilicity, ionization state, etc. ;
- Physicochemical properties of the container: nature of the material, crystallinity, porosity, thickness, nature and content of additives, etc. ;
- Container-content system operating conditions: temperature, contact time, contact surface, etc.

CCI phenomena occur in a variety of fields, including the food and pharmaceutical industries, where they can compromise product quality and consumer safety **[4]**. In the pharmaceutical sector, CCI can occur at every stage of the drug life cycle. During manufacture, packaging, storage, distribution and administration, medicines come into contact with a wide range of equipment of different natures, shapes and sizes (manufacturing equipment, packaging systems and administration devices) **[12]**. These contacts can generate CCI, among other things.

The term "container-content interactions" encompasses a range of phenomena that differ in the way they transfer substances (**Figure 1**).

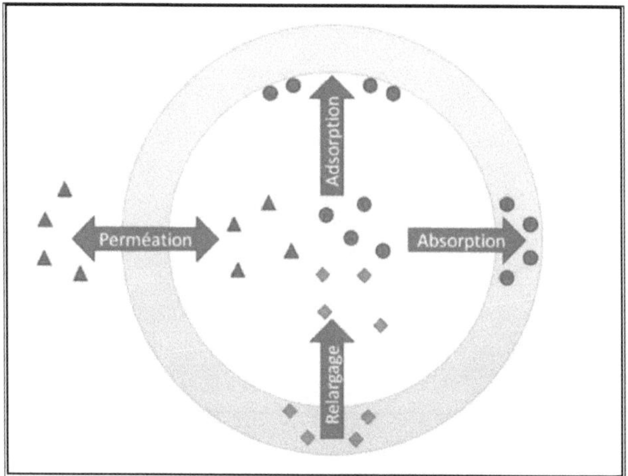


**Figure1 : The different types of container-content interactions [13]**

These phenomena are **[11]** :

- **Sorption phenomena** involve the transfer of molecules from the content to the container. Sorption is subdivided into two processes: adsorption and absorption;
- **Release phenomena** involving the migration of compounds from the container to the contents;
- **Permeation phenomena**, which concern the passage of substances through the container, whether from the contents to the outside environment or vice versa.

### 2.1.1. Adsorption

Adsorption is a surface phenomenon in which molecules (active ingredients or excipients) bind to the surface of a material (**Figure 2) [11]**. At the molecular level, there are two types of adsorption: physical adsorption, or physisorption, and chemical adsorption, or chemisorption.

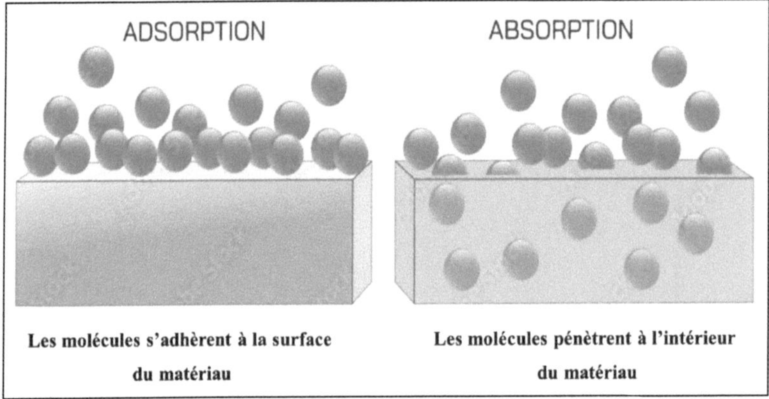


**Figure2 : Schematic representation of sorption phenomena**

During physisorption, molecules are attached to the surface of the material by low-energy interactions: Van der Waals forces and hydrogen bonds. As a result, this interaction is reversible, and adsorbed molecules can be removed from the surface by variations in temperature or pressure. Chemisorption, on the other hand, involves strong chemical bonds, often covalent, between the adsorbed molecules and those on the surface of the material, making the interaction generally irreversible.

Adsorption is also a rapid phenomenon (it can be triggered as soon as the container and contents come into contact) and saturable (once all the surface sites likely to bind molecules are occupied, no further adsorption can take place) **[11]**. The extent of this interaction depends on a number of factors, including the concentration of the active ingredient or excipient (known as the adsorbate), the available surface area and the duration of contact between the container and the contents. In addition, the pH of the contents and the pKa/pKb values of the adsorbate influence adsorption, particularly that of ionizable molecules. When conditions favor the ionized form, adsorption is facilitated on surfaces carrying an opposite charge and disadvantaged on those with the same charge as the adsorbate.

### 2.1.2. Absorption

Absorption is a physical phenomenon in which molecules (active ingredients or excipients) penetrate and diffuse within a material (**figure 2) [11]**. It follows on from adsorption, and evolves more slowly: molecules that have attached themselves to the surface then gradually penetrate the interior of the material.

Several factors influence the kinetics and extent of this phenomenon, notably the concentration of products subject to absorption, the contact time and the physico-chemical properties of the material **[11]**. The higher the concentration of molecules to be absorbed and the longer the contact time, the more significant the absorption. In addition, additives such as plasticizers, incorporated into plastics, promote this phenomenon to varying degrees. In addition, the physico-chemical properties of molecules, such as their lipophilicity, play an important role. Indeed, lipophilic molecules are more likely to be absorbed by plastics than hydrophilic molecules.

### 2.1.3. Reloading

Release is a phenomenon during which compounds initially present in the container are transferred to the contents **[14]**. These compounds, known as leachables, present a wide chemical diversity (organic and inorganic substances) and come from multiple sources **[12]**. The main categories of compounds likely to be involved in a release phenomenon are the following **[15]**:

- **Additives** for plastic and elastomer materials ;
- **Additives** for glass and metal materials ;
- Material **degradation products** (e.g. silicon from glass degradation and iron from stainless steel corrosion);
- **Residual monomers and low-molecular-weight oligomers** resulting from incomplete polymerization of plastics ;
- **Compounds from secondary and tertiary packaging**, such as printing inks and label adhesives.

In the case of a plastic material designed to contain a liquid drug, release is described by the following three phases **[16]**:

- **Diffusion within the material**: relargables move through the polymeric network in a random fashion, often obeying Fick's diffusion laws;
- **Solvatation**: at the container/content interface, relargables detach from the material and pass into the content via solvatation;
- **Dispersion within the contents**: solvated releargable molecules move away from the container/content interface and disperse within the contents. This stage is accelerated by agitation.

Moreover, the release of compounds from plastics is influenced by several factors **[1]**:

- **Release factors:** molecular weight, steric hindrance, type of bond with the material (covalent or non-covalent). The molecules most likely to be released are those that are not covalently bonded, have a low molecular weight and are structurally unobtrusive;

- **Material factors:** amorphous polymers favour the migration of molecules through their chains, while semi-crystalline polymers present barriers to migration in their crystalline zones;
- **Factors related to use:** migration increases proportionally with temperature and duration of contact.

### 2.1.4. Permeation

Permeation is the process by which molecules (of a gas or liquid) present on one side of a material, pass through the latter to emerge on the other side (this step is called desorption) **[13]**. When a material separates a drug from the outside environment, permeation may correspond either to the migration of the drug's active ingredients or excipients to the outside, or to the penetration of water vapor, oxygen, carbon dioxide or other gases from the outside environment through the material to the drug. Permeation is an irreversible phenomenon, influenced mainly by temperature and the nature of the material. Plastics and elastomers are the most favorable to this phenomenon.

## 2.2. Consequences of container-content interactions

Although the consequences of CCI often affect drugs, containers are not exempt from some of the repercussions associated with these phenomena. In fact, they can undergo the following changes **[17]** :

- Color change ;
- Modification of surface quality ;
- Increased fragility;
- Increased permeability ;
- Impaired functionality.

CCIs are dreaded phenomena by manufacturers and competent authorities alike, because of their far-reaching consequences, not only on the quality of medicines, but also on their efficacy and safety.

**2.2.1. Consequences of sorption phenomena**

Sorption of a significant quantity of active substance exposes the patient to therapeutic underdosing, which may lead to treatment failure or even deterioration in the patient's state of health **[18]**. Similarly, significant sorption of an excipient (such as an antimicrobial preservative, antioxidant, surfactant or co-solvent) deprives the drug of its effect, which may lead to instability or even loss of efficacy.

**2.2.2. Consequences of release phenomena**

Significant migration of substances from the container leads to an increase in the number of particles in the drug. This is of particular concern for parenteral products**[18]**. Similarly, relargables can alter the efficacy and stability of drugs by degrading active substances and excipients or causing them to precipitate **[19]**.

Furthermore, the most feared risk associated with salting-out is the toxicity of salts **[17]**. This toxicity may manifest itself in the short term (allergic or immunological reactions) or develop progressively (reprotoxicity, mutagenicity, carcinogenicity, etc.). Finally, migration can have other harmful consequences, such as :

- Changes in the drug's organoleptic characteristics (color, odor, taste);
- Changes in the physico-chemical parameters of the drug, such as changes in pH ;
- Analytical interference when dosing the active ingredient.

### 2.2.3. Consequences of permeation phenomena

Permeation is the main cause of drug instability **[18]**:

- Solvent loss ;
- Loss of excipients, in particular preservatives;
- Penetration of reactive gases such as oxygen and water vapor, which can degrade active ingredients or sensitive excipients (oxidation, hydrolysis, etc.).

## 3. REGULATORY REQUIREMENTS

The discovery of container-content interactions has given rise to concern among healthcare professionals and manufacturers **alike [20]**. Indeed, the impact of these interactions on drug quality, efficacy and safety has been confirmed by numerous studies. As a result, the pharmaceutical industry was forced to manage and control these interactions. To do so, they needed documents that specified the process for evaluating and controlling these phenomena. The competent authorities and the scientific community then got involved in drawing up these documents.

At present, CCI assessment and control processes are described in five categories of documents **[20]** :

- Regulatory guidelines and guides ;
- Pharmacopoeia monographs ;
- National and international standards ;
- Good practice recommendations ;
- Individual publications.

**Table III** details the properties of each category, in particular regulatory status and nature of content. Despite its diversity, international regulations are not very focused on CCIs. They often deal with "overly general concepts, leaving the technical and practical implementation of requirements open to interpretation" **[21]**. On the other hand, there is no agreement on regulatory guidelines for the assessment and control of these phenomena **[4]**. It is therefore possible to find numerous documents that are not always consistent with each other.

**TableIII : Sources of CCI assessment requirements and recommendations, according to [20].**

| Document type | Regulatory status | Nature of content |
|---|---|---|
| Regulatory guidelines and guides | Legal and mandatory requirements to obtain marketing approval for pharmaceutical products | - Contain general fuzzy application concepts;<br>- Specify what to do but not how to do it;<br>- Contain few explanations and justifications for the requirements. |
| Pharmacopoeia monographs | Legal and mandatory requirements at the discretion of the competent authorities | - Contain general fuzzy application concepts;<br>- Specify what to do and how to do it;<br>- Specify acceptance criteria;<br>- Contain few explanations and justifications for the requirements. |
| National or international standards | Legal and mandatory requirements only if recognized and adopted by the relevant authorities, otherwise recognized and adopted as consensus best practice | - Contain general fuzzy application concepts;<br>- Specify what to do but not how to do it;<br>- Contain few explanations and justifications for the requirements. |
| Best practice recommendations | Consensus opinions provided by a group of experts. Can be incorporated into regulations, standards or monographs | - Contain general concepts and specific recommended practices;<br>- Specify what to do and how to do it;<br>- Contain detailed justifications and explanations of the requirements. |
| Individual publications | Advice provided by individual experts. Can be incorporated into regulations, recommendations and monographs | - Dealing with specific subjects and situations.<br>- Can specify what to do and how to do it in these situations. |

**Table IV** lists the main international documents in which CCI assessment recommendations are discussed. In this chapter, we have discussed in detail the requirements contained in the guidelines, regulatory guides and monographs most frequently cited in the literature.

**TableIV : Main CCI evaluation documents, according to[4]**

| Document | Type | Source |
|---|---|---|
| Industry guide: container-closure systems for packaging human drugs and biological products | Regulatory guide | FDA |
| Industry guide: Nasal spray, solution, suspension and inhalation spray | Regulatory guide | FDA |
| Guideline for immediate plastic packaging materials | Guideline | EMEA |
| Pharmaceutical quality guideline for inhalation and nasal products | Guideline | EMEA |
| USP < 661 > ; < 661.1 > ; < 661.2 > ; < 1661 > ; < 660 > ; < 1660 > ; < 381 > ; < 1381 > ; < 662 > ; < 1662 > ; < 1663 > ; < 1664 > | Monographs | USP |
| 3.1.1 ; 3.1.3 ; 3.1.4 ; 3.1.5 ; 3.1.6 ; 3.1.7 ; 3.1.8 ; 3.1.9; 3.1.10 ; 3.1.11 ; 3.1.13 ; 3.1.14 ; 3.1.15 ; 3.2.1 ; 3.2.2 ; 3.2.2.1 ; 3.2.9 ; 3.3.1 ; 3.3.2 ; 3.3.3 ; 3.3.4 ; 3.3.5 ; 3.3.6 ; 3.3.7 ; 3.3.8 | Monographs | Ph. Eur. |
| ISO 8871: Elastomer parts for parenteral drugs and devices for pharmaceutical use | International standard | ISO |
| ISO 10993: Biological evaluations of medical devices | International standard | ISO |
| ICH Q3A: impurities in new drug substances | International standard | ICH |
| ICH Q3B (R2): impurities in new drugs | International standard | ICH |
| ICH Q3D: guideline on elemental impurities | International standard | ICH |
| Safety thresholds and best practices for extractables and leachables for inhalation and nasal medications | Best practice recommendations | PQRI |

**FDA:** US Food and Drug Administration; **EMEA:** European Medicines Agency; **USP:** US Pharmacopoeia; **Ph. Eur.** European Pharmacopoeia; **ISO:** International Organization for Standardization; **ICH:** International Council on Harmonization of Technical

Requirements for Registration of Pharmaceuticals for Human Use; **PQRI:** Product Quality Research Institute.

## 3.1. U.S. regulations

### 3.1.1. American Pharmacopoeia

The United States Pharmacopoeia (USP) is a compendium of standards concerning the identity, quality and safety of pharmaceutical products and their constituents. The creation of the USP dates back to the early $^{19th}$ century **[22]**. Eleven doctors, concerned about the dangers of poor-quality medicines in circulation at the time, founded an independent, non-profit scientific organization to improve public health. A year after its creation, the organization published the first edition of the USP. This described the safest medicinal substances and preparations at the time. Since then, the USP has undergone numerous modifications, culminating in its current form.

In 1906, USP standards of quality, content and purity were recognized as official by the US Food and Drug Administration **[22]**. In 1938, the U.S. Congress passed a law requiring manufacturers to test their drugs for compliance with USP standards of identity, content, safety and purity, and to submit the test results to the U.S. Food and Drug Administration (FDA) before marketing. Today, USP standards are adopted and applied by 140 countries worldwide.

#### 3.1.1.1. Terms related to container-content interactions

In the American Pharmacopoeia, several monographs have defined terms relating to pharmaceutical packaging and CCIs.

According to Monograph 659, Packaging and Storage Requirements **[23]**:

- **A container-closure system** (also called a packaging system): is the set of packaging components that contain and protect the pharmaceutical product. This includes primary and secondary CEs.
- **A container**: is a device used to hold an active substance, intermediate, excipient or finished product, and which is in direct contact with its contents (ampoules, vials, pre-filled syringes and injection pens are examples of containers).
- **A closure**: is a device used to cover the open space of a container and protect its contents. It also allows access to the container's contents (e.g. caps).
- **A packaging component**: is any element of packaging or of the container-closure system. This includes: container, closure, administration accessories, administration ports, cardboard boxes, labels, etc.
    - **Primary CE:** any CE in direct contact or which may come into direct contact with the pharmaceutical product (containers and closures).
    - **Secondary CE:** is any CE in direct contact with the primary CE and which can provide additional protection for the pharmaceutical product (e.g. cartons).
    - **Tertiary CE:** is any CE in direct contact with the secondary CE and which can provide additional protection for the pharmaceutical product during transport and/or storage (e.g. cardboard boxes).
    - **An associated component**: is any EC intended to administer the drug to the patient and which is not stored in contact with the drug

throughout its shelf life (spoons, dosing cups or caps and dosing syringes are associated packaging components).

- **Construction materials (CM):** these are the substances used to manufacture CE (glass, plastics, elastomers, metals, etc.).

According to monograph1663, entitled "Evaluation of extractables associated with pharmaceutical packaging systems" **[15]**:

- **Extractables**: organic or inorganic substances released from SE, CE or MC into extraction media. The process takes place under specific laboratory conditions (temperature, time, solvent(s), etc.).
- **Extraction study**: is the process by which extractable profiles of SEs, CEs or MCs are developed. Typically, extraction studies take place in two phases: extract generation (extraction) and extract testing (characterization).
- **The extractables profile**: is a qualitative and/or quantitative analytical representation of the substances extracted by a given solvent, under specific conditions.
- **Extraction**: is the process of exposing a material to a solvent to recover soluble substances. It is a complex process, influenced by the extraction medium (solvents), temperature, contact time, the ratio of material surface area per unit volume of solvent, and the equilibrium phase of the material.
- **Characterization**: is the process of discovering, identifying and quantifying any organic or inorganic substance present in an extract at a value above a specified level or threshold. These thresholds may be based on patient safety considerations, material considerations or the detection capabilities of the analytical techniques adopted.

According to monograph 1664, entitled "Evaluation of relargables associated with pharmaceutical packaging systems" **[12]**:

- **Relargables**: are organic or inorganic impurities found in finished products. They leach into these products from their packaging systems, under normal conditions of use and storage, or during accelerated stability studies. Relargables are generally a subset of extractables or are derivatives of extractables.
- **Relargables study**: is the process of characterizing (discovering, identifying and quantifying) the relargables that have accumulated in a drug product during its proposed shelf life.

#### 3.1.1.2.Requirements for plastic packaging systems

USP monographs "661", "661.1", "661.2" and "1661" are devoted to requirements for plastic packaging systems for pharmaceutical use and their materials of construction. According to monograph 1661, pharmaceutical products are likely to interact with plastic materials during manufacture, storage and administration **[24]**. These interactions can alter product characteristics, in particular quality, efficacy, purity and stability. Applicants for marketing authorization (MA) and manufacturers of pharmaceutical products are therefore called upon to prove that their packaging systems are chemically appropriate, i.e. that they do not interact with the products they contain in such a way as to significantly alter their characteristics. To this end, they are called upon to carry out the tests described in monographs 661.1 and 661.2, and those described in the monographs mentioned in the latter two, such as monograph 87.

In addition, Monograph 1661 states that the extent of studies evaluating packaging systems in relation to drug interactions varies according to various factors, such as the route of administration, the drug form and the nature of the material of construction (**Table V) [24].**

**Table VV : Evaluation tests for plastic packaging systems, according to [25].**

| Test name | Oral and topical forms[a] | All other shapes |
|---|---|---|
| | **Physicochemical tests** | |
| UV absorbance | X* | X* |
| Acidity / Alkalinity | X[b] | X[b] |
| Total organic carbon | X* | X* |
| Solution appearance | X* | X* |
| Total terephthaloyl fragments | PET and PET G only[c] | PET and PET G only[c] |
| Ethylene glycol | PET and PET G only[c] | PET and PET G only[c] |
| | **Biological reactivity tests** | |
| *In vitro* biological reactivity tests | ---* | X* |
| | **Chemical suitability for use** | |
| Evaluation | Risk-based testing | Risk-based testing |

X* Means test to be performed

---* Means do not perform the test

[a]For aqueous oral liquids, which contain co-solvents (or for whatever reason, the drug is likely to extract greater quantities of substances from plastic packaging components than water), additional information on extractables may be required.

[b]Means that the test must be carried out when the SE is intended to contain a liquid product or a product to be dissolved in its container before use.
[c]PET and PET G stand for polyethylene terephthalate and polyethylene terephthalate G, respectively. The terephthaloyl and ethylene glycol fragment tests are to be carried out when the SE is formed from one of these two materials.

❖ **Physico-chemical tests**

Physicochemical tests are carried out mainly on aqueous extracts of SE. These are filled with purified water, sealed and then autoclaved **[25]**. The autoclave temperature should be raised to 121°C and maintained at this level for 30 minutes (if the SE deteriorates at 121°C, a lower temperature should be used). Once heating is complete, the water should be recovered for use in the various tests.

In general, physicochemical tests enable non-specific identification of extractables from plastic SEs **[10]**. In fact, the solution appearance test highlights the presence of extractables that are not soluble in an aqueous phase, without providing any information on their identities. The acidity or alkalinity test reveals the presence of acidic or basic extractables, without revealing their identities either. The total organic carbon test reveals the presence of extractables of an organic nature. Finally, the ultraviolet absorbance test reveals the presence of extractables with aromatic or unsaturated functions in their structures, without elucidating these.

❖ ***In vitro* biological reactivity tests**

The biological reactivity tests to be carried out on plastic ES are described in Monograph 87, entitled "Biological reactivity tests, *in vitro*" **[26]**. These tests are a means of assessing the toxicity of plastic ES and the substances they release into extraction media. Nevertheless, toxicity assessment using these tests alone is often considered insufficient by the competent authorities

**[25]**. These tests are required for all pharmaceutical products, with the exception of oral and topical products. Three types of test are described: agar diffusion test, direct contact test and elution test. The choice of test(s) to be performed depends in particular on the nature of the SE and its intended use. In general, biological reactivity tests involve incubating SE (whole or in pieces), or their extracts, in vessels containing mammalian cells **[26]**. After incubation, the cellular response is evaluated and assigned a value according to its amplitude. This response consists of the degeneration and deformation of cells in contact with the ES sample or extract. **Table VI** shows the degrees of biological reactivity of the agar diffusion test and the direct contact test in relation to the cell culture result.

**TableVI : Degrees of biological reactivity for agar diffusion tests and the direct contact test, according to [26].**

| Grade | Reactivity | Description of the reactivity zone |
|---|---|---|
| 0 | No | No area* under or around the sample |
| 1 | Slight | A few degenerated or malformed cells under the sample |
| 2 | Benign | Limited area under sample and less than 0.45cm beyond sample |
| 3 | Moderate | The zone extends from 0.45 to 1.0cm beyond the sample. |
| 4 | Severe | The zone extends more than 1.0cm beyond the sample. |

*cell culture inhibition zone

**Table VII** shows the degrees of biological reactivity of the elution test. In any case, SEs or their extracts should not induce cellular responses beyond grade 2.

**TableVII : Degrees of biological reactivity of elution tests, according to [26].**

| Grade | Reactivity | Description of the reactivity zone |
|---|---|---|
| 0 | No | Discrete intracytoplasmic granules; no cell lysis |
| 1 | Slight | Up to 20% of cells are rounded, weakly attached and without intracytoplasmic granules; occasional lysed cells are present. |
| 2 | Benign | Between 20% and 50% of cells are rounded and devoid of intracytoplasmic granules; no extensive cell lysis or empty areas between cells |
| 3 | Moderate | Between 50% and 70% of cell layers contain rounded or lysed cells |
| 4 | Severe | Almost complete destruction of cell layers |

❖ **Assessment of chemical suitability for use**

According to monograph 661.2, assessment of chemical fitness for use is a process that should be considered by pharmaceutical manufacturers when the risk of interactions deleterious to product quality and/or patient health is high **[25]**. This is the case, for example, with inhalation products. These products often contain active substances dissolved or dispersed in organic solvents. The latter promote the release of additives from plastic SEs **[27]**. On the other hand, drugs intended for inhalation are specifically designed for patients who are vulnerable due to alterations in their respiratory systems. Consequently, these products must be assessed for their chemical suitability for use.

The evaluation process includes **[25]**:

- Characterization of materials of construction for packaging systems using the tests described in monograph 661.1;
- Extraction studies carried out on packaging systems;
- Release studies carried out on finished products.

Extraction and salting-out studies have not been addressed in the US Pharmacopoeia by tests specifying their procedures and acceptance criteria, due to the wide diversity of packaging systems and pharmaceutical products. However, two general monographs, 1663 and 1664, have been reserved to set out the principles of these studies and provide recommendations on their proper conduct.

#### 3.1.1.3.Requirements for elastomer packaging components

Monographs 381 and 1381 are devoted to requirements for elastomer components of container-closure systems for injectable medicines (vials, pre-filled syringes, cartridges, etc.) **[28]**. Examples of these components include stoppers, seals, tip caps and needle guards. As with plastic CEs, those made from elastomers should not interact with pharmaceutical products in a way that could jeopardize their quality and performance attributes (efficacy, purity, stability, etc.).

Monograph 381 describes the tests that should be carried out on elastomer CEs to prove this. As with plastic CEs, these tests include: physicochemical tests, biological reactivity tests, extraction studies and salting-out studies **[28]**. The procedures and acceptance criteria for physicochemical tests are specified in Monograph 381, while those for biological reactivity tests are specified in Monographs 87 and 88.

### 3.1.2. Guide to packaging systems for drugs and biological products

The SE Guide for Drugs and Biologics is an official document published in 1999 in the USA. It was developed by the Packaging Technical Committee at the Center for Drug Evaluation and Research, in collaboration with the FDA's Center for Biologics Evaluation and Research **[19]**. This guide replaces the FDA's 1987 guidance on the submission of packaging documents for drugs and biological products, as well as the packaging policy statement published by the Office of Generic Drugs in 1995.

This guide is also intended for manufacturers. Its aim is to make them aware of the FDA's requirements concerning the quality of pharmaceutical packaging, and the data they should include in their drug registration dossiers to prove this quality and guarantee its preservation for all batches to be produced **[19]**. For this reason, manufacturers wishing to market new pharmaceutical products are invited to apply the provisions of this guide. Nevertheless, any approach other than that proposed by this guide is permitted, but is likely to be rejected by the FDA.

According to the guide, pharmaceutical packaging should have four essential properties **[19]**. It should :

- Protect the pharmaceutical product properly;
- Be compatible with the pharmaceutical product;
- Constructed of safe materials;
- Function correctly.

On the other hand, through this guide, the FDA has proposed the classification of drugs into categories using two criteria: the probability of

CCI and the degree of concern associated with the route of administration. The choice of these two criteria is based on experimental data which reported that:

- The probability of CCI is closely linked to the form of the pharmaceutical product. Products in liquid form are more likely to interact with their packaging than products in solid form;
- The health risk posed by CCIs depends on the route of administration. Parenteral, ophthalmic and inhalation routes are considered the most critical, unlike oral and topical routes.

**Table VIII** shows the different categories of pharmaceutical products classified according to the two above-mentioned criteria. This classification forms the basis for various requirements in the guide. Indeed, the higher the probability of CCI and the more critical the route of administration, the more stringent the requirements on packaging quality and on the tests to be carried out and data to be submitted to prove this quality.

**TableVIII : Drug classification according to the FDA concept, based on[19].**

| **Degree of concern associated with route of administration** | **Probability of container-content interactions** | | |
|---|---|---|---|
| | **High** | **Average** | **Low** |
| **Very high** | Aerosols and inhalation solutions; injections and suspensions* for injection | Sterile powders and powders for injection; powders for inhalation | |

| | | | |
|---|---|---|---|
| **High** | Ophthalmic solutions and suspensions*; ointments and transdermal devices; aerosols and nasal sprays | | |
| **Low** | Topical solutions and suspensions*; topical and lingual aerosols; oral solutions and suspensions*. | Topical powders; oral powders | Tablets and capsules |

Suspensions*: for the purposes of this table, the term suspension refers to any pharmaceutical preparation formed from two immiscible phases (a solid in a liquid, or a liquid in a liquid). It therefore covers a broad category of products: creams, emulsions, gels and suspensions in the pharmaceutical sense.

In this guide, requirements relating to CCIs are mainly to be found in section III, reserved for the qualification and quality control of packaging, and in particular in the paragraphs dealing with protection, compatibility and safety.

#### 3.1.2.1.Protection

Packaging for pharmaceutical use must protect its contents from factors likely to degrade its quality, from manufacture to expiry date **[19]**.

These factors are:

- Light exposure;
- Exposure to reactive gases such as oxygen;
- Water vapour absorption ;
- Solvent loss ;
- Microbial contamination.

Moreover, sensitivity to these factors differs from one product to another. Some products are photosensitive and/or degrade in the presence of humidity. Others, on the other hand, retain their quality in the presence of these factors. Consequently, manufacturers are advised to carry out studies on their products to determine which of these factors have a major influence on their qualities. They are then required to assess the protection afforded by their packaging against potential factors, and to report the results of this assessment in their drug registration files. To this end, pharmaceutical laboratories can carry out USP tests where they exist, such as the light transmission test, which assesses the protection of packaging against light transmission. Where appropriate, other tests can be carried out, provided that the competent authorities are supplied with their interest, validation and operating procedures.

In general, any packaging for a photosensitive product, regardless of its galenic form, should protect it from light **[19]**. Packaging for liquid products should protect them from solvent loss. Packaging for sterile products (injectables, ophthalmics) should protect against microbial contamination. Protection against water vapor penetration concerns solid pharmaceutical forms (powders, tablets, capsules). Finally, guaranteeing against the penetration of reactive gases is essentially reserved for liquid products administered parenterally, ophthalmically and by inhalation.

#### 3.1.2.2.Compatibility

Compatibility is defined in this guide as the absence of a harmful interaction between the drug and its SE that may lead to degradation of the quality of one or the other **[19]**. Examples of such interactions include:

- Reduced efficacy of the drug due to sorption of the active substance or its degradation by a substance extracted from the SE ;
- Reduction in excipient concentration due to sorption or degradation;
- Changes in the color of the drug or SE ;
- Modification of the drug's pH ;
- The rush;
- Increased SE fragility.

In some cases, CCIs only become apparent after a long period of contact between the pharmaceutical product and its packaging **[19]**. It is therefore recommended that during stability studies, manufacturers investigate any changes in quality which may be attributable to CCI, and take the necessary steps to correct them.

On the other hand, compatibility between packaging and pharmaceutical products depends essentially on the drug form:

- Liquid forms are the most susceptible to incompatibilities;
- Solid forms intended to be reconstituted in appropriate solvents just before use, present risks of interactions after reconstitution;
- Solid forms intended to be administered as they present the least risk of interactions.

In addition, to prove the compatibility of packaging with its contents, US Pharmacopoeia tests on pharmaceutical packaging are often sufficient.

#### 3.1.2.3.Security

In the guide, packaging safety is defined by the use of CTs that do not transfer harmful substances or high quantities of impurities to the pharmaceutical product **[19]**. This property is essential for CEs in direct contact with the product (primary CEs). However, it must be present in all other components from which substances can migrate to the product, such as inks or adhesives. To demonstrate the safety of packaging, manufacturers are required to indicate the full chemical composition of the product, and to adopt one of the following processes, depending on the product category:

- For inhalation products, an exhaustive study is recommended. First, an extraction study must be carried out, followed by a toxicological evaluation to characterize (identify and quantify) the substances likely to migrate into the drug, and assess their potential toxicity. Secondly, extractable levels must be monitored for each batch of product;
- For injectable and ophthalmic drugs, compliance with USP specifications for biological reactivity (for plastic and elastomer packaging) and hydrolytic resistance (for glass packaging) is often sufficient. Otherwise, an extraction study followed by a toxicological evaluation may be more appropriate;
- For other medicines, the use of construction materials approved under food packaging regulations is generally considered sufficient proof of packaging safety.

## 3.2. European regulations

### 3.2.1. European Pharmacopoeia

The European Pharmacopoeia (Ph. Eur.) is a scientific and technical work whose contents fall within the pharmaceutical field. It defines the quality and safety criteria to be met by medicines and their ingredients, and details the tests used to demonstrate these criteria. The decision to draw up a Ph. Eur. dates back to 1964, when 8 European countries (Belgium, France, Germany, Italy, Luxembourg, the Netherlands, Switzerland and the United Kingdom) signed a convention on the harmonization of specifications relating to medicinal substances and pharmaceutical preparations, to facilitate their circulation and distribution in Europe **[29]**. Since then, several European countries have joined the Ph. Eur. development convention, to form a community of 38 members **[30]**.Ph. Eur. texts are classified into three categories: general chapters, general monographs and specific monographs. The general chapters cover analytical methods, reagents, materials used in the manufacture of vessels and containers, and other miscellaneous topics. Monographs cover pharmaceutical products (radiopharmaceutical preparations, vaccines, immunosera, homeopathic products, etc.), active substances, excipients, etc.

Unless otherwise specified, Ph. Eur. monographs (general and specific) constitute official technical rules of mandatory application in the territories of the contracting states **[30]**. General chapters, on the other hand, only constitute mandatory requirements if a monograph refers to them.

In the Ph. Eur. the CCIs were dealt with either implicitly or vaguely, leaving readers free to interpret the texts and devise their own evaluation methods. This subject has been dealt with in general chapter number three, entitled "Materials used in the manufacture of containers and receptacles".

This chapter is subdivided into three sub-chapters in the following order:

- 3.1: Materials used in the manufacture of containers ;
- 3.2 : Containers ;
- 3.3: Containers for human blood and blood components, and materials used in their manufacture; transfusion sets and materials used in their manufacture; syringes.

#### 3.2.1.1.Requirements of subchapter 3.1

This sub-chapter of the Ph. Eur. is essentially dedicated to polymers used in the manufacture of packaging and some medical devices (parenteral nutrition tubing). The polymers listed are plasticized and unplasticized polyvinyl chloride, polyethylene (with and without additives), polyethylene vinyl acetate, polyolefins, polypropylene and polyethylene terephthalate. For each polymer, the Ph.Eur. specifies the following points **[31]** :

- **Intended use**: polymer intended for the manufacture of containers for parenteral preparations, polymer intended for the manufacture of containers for ophthalmic preparations, etc. ;
- **Qualitative and quantitative composition**: nature of monomers and additives and their respective contents;
- **Polymer identification and characterization tests**: polymer identification by infrared absorption spectrophotometry, additive identification by chromatographic methods, polymer characterization by the following tests: solution appearance, absorbency, acidity or alkalinity, reducing substances, extractable elements, etc.

This section does not explicitly address the subject of ICC. It can be deduced from the following provisions **[31]** :

- Fixing polymer formulations: for example, polyethylene for parenteral and ophthalmic containers must be obtained either by polymerizing ethylene in the presence of catalysts, or by copolymerizing ethylene with a maximum of 25% higher homologous alkenes ($C_3$ to $C_{10}$).
- Setting the nature and content of additives: taking the example of ethylene intended for the manufacture of containers for parenteral and ophthalmic preparations, this should contain as additives: a maximum of three

antioxidants, one or more lubricants or anti-blockers, and titanium dioxide as an opacifier (if the product to be packaged in it is photosensitive). In addition, the additives to be used should be selected from the Ph. Eur. list, in compliance with the levels indicated therein;

- Fixing the content of extractable elements (aluminum, chromium, titanium, zinc, etc.) from polymers;
- Manufacturers wishing to use polymers and additives other than those specified in the pharmacopoeia are required to obtain prior approval from the competent authorities;
- Manufacturers using polymers mentioned in the pharmacopoeia are required to guarantee that all batches to be produced comply with pharmacopoeia specifications.

#### 3.2.1.2.Requirements of subchapter 3.2

The "Containers" sub-chapter covers glass and plastic containers for pharmaceutical use, and rubber closures for parenteral containers. Identification and characterization tests for each category are detailed.

As far as CCIs are concerned, they are covered only by the following requirements **[8]**:

- Containers and closures for pharmaceutical use, if they release substances into medicines, must not be in quantities so high as to alter the stability of the medicines or cause toxic effects;
- Pharmaceutical containers and closures, if permeable or if they adsorb or absorb drug constituents, must do so insignificantly;

- Manufacturers of containers and closures must guarantee to drug manufacturers the reproducibility of the production process, i.e. there must be no change in the composition or properties of the containers (compared to the standard samples);
- Drug manufacturers should carry out container-content compatibility tests to prove the absence of deleterious CCI. These tests include looking for pH changes, assessing losses or gains due to possible permeability of the container or closure, biological tests, chemical tests, etc.

#### 3.2.1.3.Requirements of subchapter 3.3

This sub-chapter presents the quality and safety requirements for three types of products:

- Containers for human blood and blood components: polymer bags and bottles;
- Transfusion sets: tubing, blood filter, drip chamber, etc. ;
- Single-use plastic syringes.

The following provisions are dedicated to CCIs **[32]**:

- The materials chosen for the manufacture of containers for human blood and blood components must protect them from gas exchange and from the release of substances that may cause abnormal changes in the blood or be toxic to patients;
- The composition of transfusion sets is such as to ensure the absence of hemolytic effects.
- The inks, glues and adhesives used to mark the syringes must not migrate through the wall and contaminate the contents. In addition, if the inner

wall of the syringes is coated with a layer of silicone oil, there must be no excess which could contaminate the product.

### 3.2.2. Guideline for immediate plastic packaging

The guideline on immediate plastic packaging materials is a technical guide drawn up by the European Medicines Agency, in consultation with the competent authorities of the member states of the European Union **[33]**. Published in 2005, this guideline specifies the documents that must be attached to MA dossiers, in particular those relating to primary plastic packaging for active substances and finished products. It also sets out the general principles of CCI evaluation studies.

In this guideline, CCIs are covered in sections four, five and six, devoted respectively to extraction studies, interaction studies and toxicological documentation, as well as in appendices I and II.

#### 3.2.2.1. Extraction studies

In this section, the guideline specifies that **[34]**:

- The aim of the extraction studies is to characterize (identify and quantify) the additives in materials made of plastics that are likely to be extracted by drugs and active substances;
- Extraction studies involve exposing a sample of the packaging material to a suitable solvent under stress conditions, to increase the extraction rate. The solvent used must have an extraction power similar to that of the active substance or drug in question;
- The need for extraction studies depends on a number of factors: the route of administration, the drug form, the description of the material in Ph. Eur. and the approval of the material by food packaging regulations.

Extraction studies are required for materials not described in Ph. Eur. and intended for the manufacture of containers for non-solid parenteral, ophthalmic or inhalation drugs. Extraction studies are also required for packaging materials for active substances and non-solid oral and topical medicinal products when these materials are not described in either the Ph. Eur. or food packaging regulations.

#### 3.2.2.2.Interaction studies

Interaction studies are used to assess container-content compatibility **[34]**. Their scope and design depend essentially on the drug form. Drugs and active substances in solid forms do not require interaction studies (drugs in solid forms intended for parenteral or inhalation administration, such as lyophilisates, may, however, require interaction studies), given the low risk of ICC phenomena occurring with these forms. For active substances and drugs in liquid form, the risk of CCI is high, so interaction studies are required. These studies should demonstrate that no significant alteration in the quality of the pharmaceutical product has occurred as a result of CHF. Interaction studies include migration and sorption studies.

With regard to migration studies, the guide clarifies the following points **[34]**:

- Migration studies should be carried out during drug development, to enable the selection of safe packaging materials;
- They are required when extraction studies result in one or more extractables whose concentrations are not low enough to present no risk to the efficacy, stability and safety of the product;

- They should be carried out on at least one batch of active substance or medicinal product;
- They are carried out by exposing the final material/packaging to the active substance/drug, under normal conditions of storage and use. If the packaging consists of overlapping films of different plastic materials, the migration of substances from the outer layers into the product should be assessed, depending on the nature of the product and its intended use. In addition, it must be demonstrated that the ink or adhesives applied to the outside of the packaging do not transfer any substances into the drug.

With regard to sorption studies, the guideline specifies that **[34]**:

- Sorption studies may be considered during drug development to investigate possible alterations in drug quality due to sorption of an active substance or excipient;
- They are mandatory when stability studies have led to a change in the quality of the drug that may be attributable to sorption of one or more constituents.

#### 3.2.2.3. Toxicological documentation

Toxicological data on substances detected during extraction and migration studies should be attached to marketing authorization dossiers, according to their chemical structure and content **[34]**.

#### 3.2.2.4. Appendices I and II

Appendices I and II of the guideline (reproduced here in **Tables IX, X** and **XI**) are decision trees.

These specify the studies that should be carried out for a plastic material/packaging (extraction study, migration study, sorption study) and the documents that should be attached to MA dossiers (general information, specifications, toxicological data), depending on the form of drug/active substance, route of administration and other criteria.

**TableIX : Plastic packaging materials for active substances**

| Documents | Solid active substance | Non-solid active substance | |
|---|---|---|---|
| | | Condition 1* | Condition 2* |
| **General information** | Yes | Yes | Yes |
| **Specifications** | Yes | Yes | Yes |
| **Extraction studies** | No | No | Yes |
| **Migration studies** | No | Yes | Yes |
| **Toxicological documentation** | No | No | Yes |

*General information: information on the materials used in the manufacture of packaging, such as the chemical name of the material, the chemical name(s) of the monomers making up the material, the name of the supplier and the qualitative composition of the material, including additives.

*Specifications: description of the material and its mechanical and physical properties, results of material identification test(s), results of tests to identify the main additives, etc. These tests are those of the European Pharmacopoeia or are established by the supplier in compliance with the Ph.Eur. methodology when a monograph describing the material is not available either in the Ph.Eur. or in a pharmacopoeia. These tests are those of the European Pharmacopoeia, or are established by the supplier using the Ph.Eur.

methodology when a monograph describing the material is not available either in the Ph.Eur. or in a member state pharmacopoeia.

*Condition 1: the plastic material is described in the Ph. Eur. or in a member state pharmacopoeia and/or is included in food packaging legislation.

*Condition 2: the plastic material is not described in either the Ph. Eur. or a member state pharmacopoeia, and is not included in food packaging legislation.

**Table XX : Plastic packaging materials for oral and topical medications**

| Documentation | Solid shapes | Non-solid forms | |
|---|---|---|---|
| | | Condition 1* | Condition 2* |
| **General information** | Yes | Yes | Yes |
| **Specifications** | Yes | Yes | Yes |
| **Extraction studies** | No | No | Yes |
| **Interaction studies** | No | Yes | Yes |
| **Toxicological information** | No | No | Yes |

*Condition 1: the plastic material is described in the Ph. Eur. or in a member state pharmacopoeia and/or is included in food packaging legislation.

*Condition 2: the plastic material is not described in either the Ph. Eur. or a member state pharmacopoeia, and is not included in food packaging legislation.

**TableXI : Plastic packaging materials for injectables, ophthalmics and inhalants**

| Documentation | Solid shapes | Non-solid forms | |
|---|---|---|---|
| | | Condition 1* | Condition 2* |

| **General information** | Yes | Yes | Yes |
|---|---|---|---|
| **Specifications** | Yes | Yes | Yes |
| **Extraction studies** | No | No | Yes |
| **Interaction studies** | Yes (if required) | Yes | Yes |
| **Toxicological information** | No | No | Yes |

*Condition 1: the plastic material is described in the Ph. Eur. or in a member state pharmacopoeia and/or is included in food packaging legislation.
*Condition 2: the plastic material is not described in either the Ph. Eur. or a member state pharmacopoeia, and is not included in food packaging legislation.

# 4. CASE STUDIES

In the pharmaceutical sector, container-content interactions can occur in three types of situation **[20]**:

- **During the drug manufacturing process:** raw materials and intermediate products pass through a variety of equipment (mixers, filters, filling machines, etc.) before being transformed into finished products. These different phases can give rise to CCIs;
- **During drug storage:** once manufactured, drugs are packaged in SEs until they are used. During this phase, CCIs are considered;
- **During drug administration:** some galenic forms are administered to patients using appropriate medical devices, which can cause CCI.

## 4.1. Interactions between pharmaceutical products and manufacturing equipment

Drug manufacturing equipment is made up of stainless steel parts. Although this material was once considered inert, it has certain drawbacks **[20]**. In addition to the risk of cross-contamination, these installations are complex, and their cleaning, sterilization and maintenance stages are time-consuming and costly **[9]**. This has led to the design and development of sterile single-use equipment (also known as disposable equipment), mainly made of plastics.

Gradually, this new equipment invaded the pharmaceutical industry, particularly the biologics industry. Although they have overcome the failures of older installations, their use has increased the number of CCI incidents **[20]**.

The disposable equipment commonly used in the production of biological drugs includes filters, tubing, connectors and finally bags, which are the most involved in CCI phenomena **[9]**. Used for ingredient mixing, sampling, storage and transportation, bags have gradually replaced conventional bioreactors.

On the other hand, pouches are multi-layers formed by superimposed films of distinct plastic materials, each of which imparts a specific physico-chemical property to the whole **[9]**. While the outer layer ensures durability and impact resistance, the inner film, intended to be in direct contact with the drugs and their constituents, is generally made of low-molecular-weight polyethylene, used as the first choice given its excellent chemical compatibility profile. In addition, to facilitate processing and increase the stability of these polymers, other additives such as slip agents and antioxidants are often added **[9]**. Slip agents lubricate the inner walls of the pouches, thus preventing adhesion. Antioxidants prevent degradation of the pouches by atmospheric oxygen or during production (high temperatures) and processing (sterilization by ionizing radiation). Nevertheless, these additives and their degradation products are liable to migrate from the films and infiltrate the product in contact**[9]**. At this level, they can degrade product quality, compromising efficacy, safety and the manufacturing process.

Hammond et *al.*, in a study of Chinese hamster ovary (CHO) cell culture in six single-use bioreactors from different suppliers (A, B, C, D, E and F), reported the identification of a chemical substance from the pouch-forming material, which caused cell culture damage **[35]**.

To analyze this event, identical cell culture media were incubated in the pouches for 3 days at 37°C. CHO cells were then seeded in 24-well plates, using the same culture media. After incubation, live cells were counted using a cytometer. The authors found that, in three of the six culture media (bioreactors A, B and F), cell density was significantly reduced compared with the control (cells grown in culture media not incubated in the bioreactors).

Secondly, extractions were carried out to identify any substance responsible for the cytotoxic effect observed **[35]**. Pieces of the disposable pouches were exposed to water at 50°C for 48 hours. The extracts were then analyzed by high-performance liquid chromatography (HPLC).

The results obtained enabled the detection of bis (2,4-di-tert-butylphenyl) phosphate (bDtBPP) in three extracts from the same pockets A, B and F. This molecule is a degradation product of tris (2,4-di-tert-butylphenyl) phosphite (known under the trade name Irgafos168) **[36]**. It is a secondary antioxidant added to polymers to protect them from degradation. It acts by deactivating hydroperoxides, reactive chemical compounds that can form when polymers are processed at very high temperatures, or during their sterilization by ionizing radiation.

This study concluded that bDtBPP, the degradation product of Irgafos 168, can migrate from the walls of disposable bioreactors and infiltrate cell cultures. At this level, it exerts a cytotoxic effect on CHO cells, inhibiting their growth even at low concentrations (0.1 mg/L) **[36]**.

In conclusion, the release of cytotoxic compounds into cell culture media represents a major risk for the production of biological drugs, particularly recombinant proteins from CHO cells **[35]**. This phenomenon prompts manufacturers to systematically assess the level of bDtBPP release from disposable bioreactors before launching recombinant protein production.

This assessment is crucial to guarantee the safety and viability of cell cultures and to ensure the quality of final products.

## 4.2. Interactions between drugs and packaging

### 4.2.1. General cases

#### 4.2.1.1. The glass

Glass is a relatively inert material **[5]**. It is compatible with most chemicals, enabling it to be used in the packaging of many types of medicine. In addition, it is distinguished by its barrier properties. It prevents the penetration of atmospheric gases (such as oxygen and water vapor) inside the container. This protects pharmaceutical products from potential degradation through oxidation or hydrolysis. Glass also prevents volatile substances from escaping into the atmosphere. As a result, drug stability and efficacy are maintained. However, glass can be involved in ICCs of its own **[5]**. In fact, glass for pharmaceutical use is formed from silica dioxide to which are added various quantities of other oxides, such as sodium, calcium, boron, aluminum, magnesium and iron oxides. With the exception of boron oxide, which establishes strong bonds with silica dioxide, the other oxides are weakly bound to the latter, allowing them to migrate freely within the glass's structural network. As a result, certain glass components can be released into the contents. For example, sodium oxide can migrate from the glass surface into aqueous solutions. The release takes place via an ion exchange process, during which hydrogen ions (from the solution) bind to the glass in place of alkali ions ($Na^+$ , $K^+$ ). As a result, the pH of the contents increases.

In addition, glass can undergo a phenomenon known as delamination **[5]**. According to the USP, delamination of glass packaging consists in the appearance of fine glass lamellae in the drug solution, ranging in size from less than 50µm to 200µm **[7]**. The appearance of lamellae is a late indicator of a strong corrosion interaction between the drug and the inner surface of the glass. This interaction involves hydrolysis and ion exchange mechanisms **[8]**. This process is favored by several factors, namely the presence of buffers in the drug solution (such as citrate and phosphate), the ionic strength of the drug solution, and the manufacturing, sterilization and end-treatment processes of glass containers.

#### 4.2.1.2.Plastics

Plastics are the materials most involved in CCI. Sorption, release and permeation can all occur with these materials to varying degrees. In the case of sorption, PVC bags have been the most incriminated. This phenomenon has affected a range of drugs, notably insulin, diazepam, amiodarone and isosorbide dinitrate**[11]**. Process residues, residual monomers and additives are all susceptible to release. However, the release of plasticizers from PVC bags is the phenomenon most widely reported in the literature.

#### 4.2.1.3.Elastomers

Like plastics, elastomers are very much involved in CCIs **[5]**. They can be permeable to gases and moisture; they can adsorb or absorb components from the contents (preservatives are known to have a high tendency to sorb to elastomer components), and synthetic residues and additives can migrate from these materials into products in contact (2-mercaptobenzothiazole, aluminum, nitrosamines and zinc are the leachables commonly found with elastomer components) **[37]**.

### 4.2.2. Interaction of a preservative with pre-filled syringes

Water for injection is the diluent of choice for parenteral drugs. For low-volume multidose forms, these may also contain antimicrobial preservatives **[38]**. These are added in minute quantities to maintain the microbiological stability of the reconstituted preparation until it is administered.

Benzyl alcohol (BzOH), packaged in glass vials, is widely used as a diluent for protein lyophilisates. However, some manufacturers have recently opted to package it in pre-filled syringes (**figure 3**).

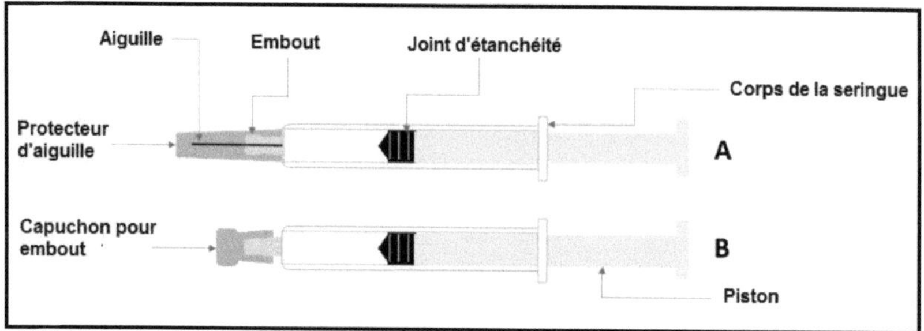


**Figure3 : Schematic representation of prefilled syringes [38].**
(A) needle syringe ;
(B) needleless syringe.

In a recent study on this subject, Thakare et *al*. reported that the concentration of BzOH decreased after 3 months during their stability study**[38]**. This finding prompted them to investigate further the phenomenon involved in the loss of the preservative. Using the Ishikawa diagram, they analyzed all the possible causes of this incident (**figure 4**).

Initially, the authors excluded causes related to measurement errors, analytical method, labor, environment, polymerization and BzOH degradation (lack of detection of degradation products, notably benzaldehyde and benzoic acid).

Consequently, the hypotheses could be related to the adhesion of BzOH to :

- ✓ Syringe body ;
- ✓ Gasket ;
- ✓ End cap.

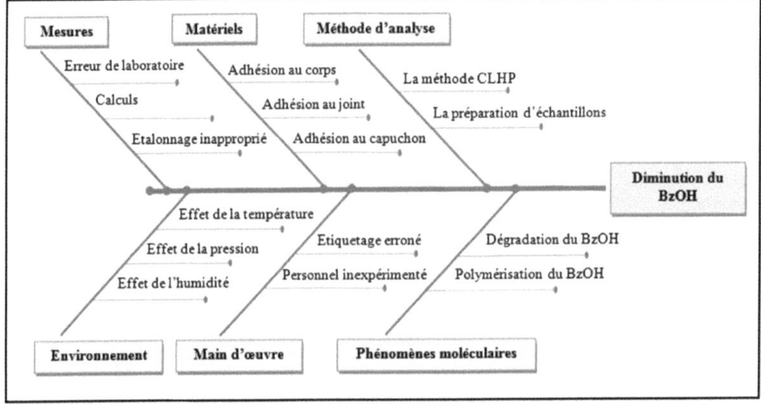


**Figure4 : Possible causes of benzyl alcohol loss, after [38]**

In order to assess possible adhesion of BzOH to the syringe body, and more specifically to the silicone oil layer applied/sprayed on its inner surface, both products were incubated for four weeks at 40°C. A weekly sample of the diluent was then taken and its BzOH concentration determined by HPLC. The results showed that the concentration was stable throughout the experiment. The first hypothesis was therefore ruled out.

In a second step, the team analyzed the possibility of interaction between the diluent and the syringe seal. Operating under the same conditions, the authors reported a non-significant decrease in the concentration of BzOH in

the diluent. In fact, although elastomers are known for their ability to adsorb preservatives, they were previously coated with a fluoropolymer layer, which helped to limit the adsorption phenomenon.
Finally, the team continued its investigation and tested the last hypothesis using the same experimental protocol. Knowing that mouthpiece caps are manufactured from elastomers without fluoropolymer surface treatment, HPLC analyses of the samples showed that the concentration of BzOH after four weeks decreased significantly (by around 15%). Thus, they concluded that the loss of the product was attributed to its adsorption on the caps **[38]**. They also demonstrated that the extent of this interaction depended on the nature of the elastomer used. Indeed, the amount of BzOH lost varied from one syringe to another, simply by changing the nature of the elastomer. Other factors also influence this phenomenon: the duration of diluent/cap contact, storage temperature, and the possible absence of the fluoropolymer layer covering the cap.
Admittedly, the addition of preservatives to multi-dose formulations can inhibit microbial proliferation, but such adsorption phenomena could have harmful consequences for both the product (loss of efficacy, altered stability, compromised safety) and the patient (risk of infection). This underlines the importance of rigorous formulation and careful control of interactions between drugs and their packaging during the R&D phase.

### 4.2.3. Moxifloxacin eye drops

Moxifloxacin (MM = 401.43 Da) is a quinolone antibiotic mainly prescribed for the treatment of bacterial conjunctivitis **[39]**.
In a stability study conducted by Gollapalli on this molecule in eye drops, an impurity was detected at 0.3% (w/w) after 24 months' storage under normal

conditions of use [40]. The identification of this impurity had not yet been established, despite an extensive literature search. The author also reported that the UV spectrum of this impurity was similar to that of moxifloxacin, suggesting that it originated from the active substance. Furthermore, this impurity was undetectable in the forced degradation study involving the active substance and the reconstituted pharmaceutical form. This finding ruled out the hypothesis that this impurity originated from the degradation of moxifloxacin.

Faced with this situation, researchers began a study to identify this new impurity and elucidate its formation process.

Initially, they used quadrupole time-of-flight liquid chromatography-mass spectrometry (LC-MS) to determine its molar mass (474.2034) and suggest its chemical formula ($C_{24}H_{28}FN_3O_6$).

Secondly, the authors attempted to determine the origin of this impurity. The first hypothesis suggesting the possibility of interaction of the active substance or one of its degradation products with another chemical compound present in the drug matrix (excipients) was ruled out. Next, they conducted an extraction study to evaluate moxifloxacin's primary packaging system, consisting of a low-molecular-weight polyethylene bottle and cap. Samples of the primary packaging components were exposed to three different extraction solvents: pH 3 buffer (sodium phosphate), pH 9 buffer (sodium bicarbonate) and ethanol/water mixture (40:60 v/v), at 50°C for 4 days. LC-MS and GC-MS analysis of these extracts detected the ethylene glycol monoformate ($C_3H_6O_3$, 90.078 Da) used in the flask composition.

In order to verify the possible involvement of this molecule in the formation of the impurity in question, the authors compared the analyses of a solution of moxifloxacin overloaded with ethylene glycol monoformate with those of a control, after contact with the bottle for one month.

The results showed that the impurity studied was absent in the control solution, unlike that containing ethylene glycol monoformate. Similarly, its quantity was proportional to the contact time.

Finally, using liquid chromatography coupled with tandem mass spectrometry, Gollapalliet *al.* were able to confirm the chemical formula of the impurity studied and elucidate its structure (**Figure 5**).

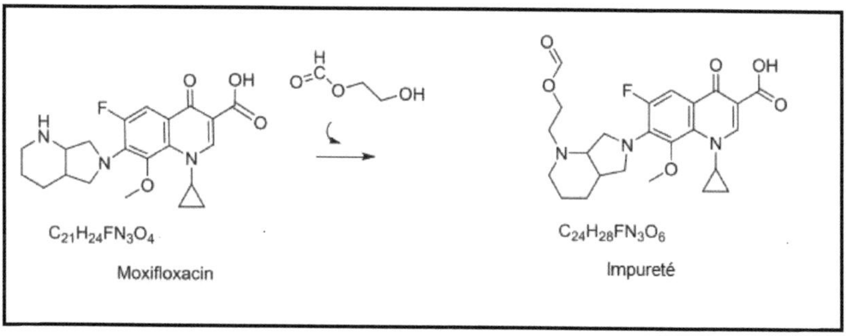

$C_{21}H_{24}FN_3O_4$ Moxifloxacin → $C_{24}H_{28}FN_3O_6$ Impureté

**Figure5 : Structure and proposed formula of the impurity, after [40].**

In this study of moxifloxacin eye drops, the researchers demonstrated the release of a reactive chemical compound (ethylene glycol monoformate) from the primary packaging (polyethylene). This compound interacted with the active substance, leading to the formation of a previously unidentified impurity. This impurity features an aldehyde group in its structure, raising concerns about drug safety and patient security.

In addition to related substances and degradation products, the purity of drugs should therefore be assessed for the presence of releasables resulting from the interaction between content and container **[41]**

### 4.2.4. Cases of antibody-mediated PRCA

PRCA is a severe normocytic normochromic anemia, hereditary or acquired **[42]**. Sporadic cases were reported in the early 1990s in patients with chronic kidney disease (CKD) **[43]**. Since then, the number of cases detected has risen considerably from 1998 onwards, reaching a peak in 2002.

The first investigations carried out suspected epoetin alfa, a recombinant protein synthesized by CHO cells, structurally identical to the human hormone (erythropoietin), which mimics its action and stimulates the production of red blood cells in the bone marrow. Indeed, the patients who developed the disease had previously received this molecule, in particular the Janssen laboratory's EPREX® speciality **[43]**. In addition, pharmacological studies have confirmed that taking this speciality has a positive effect on bone marrow production.

Induces an immunological reaction resulting in the synthesis of anti-erythropoietin antibodies **[43]**. These antibodies neutralize not only the epoetin drug, but also endogenous erythropoietin, leading to a severe reduction in medullary red blood cell precursors and thus causing anemia. This side effect has been termed "antibody-mediated erythroblastopenia" (EMA).

On the other hand, investigations into the manufacturing procedure of EPREX® (packaged in pre-filled syringes or glass vials) have been initiated with the aim of explaining the immunogenicity of this drug **[44]**. HPLC analysis of the finished product revealed the presence of additional peaks that corresponded neither to the active substance, nor to the excipients, nor to their degradation products. Mass spectrometry was used to detect organic substances that had migrated from the seals of the pre-filled syringes. The investigators suggested that this phenomenon might be promoted by polysorbate 80, a stabilizing excipient known for its ability to promote the release of substances from plastics and elastomers. Indeed, polysorbate has been included in the formulation of EPREX® since 1998, when cases of PRCA began to rise sharply.

Based on the results obtained, Boven et *al.* decided to carry out a retrospective study of reported cases of erythroblastopenia during the period from January 1'1989 to June 30, 2004, with the aim of confirming these hypotheses **[43]**. Following collection of formulation-related data from the manufacturer, and reports of this adverse event from physicians, pharmacists and patients who developed the EMA, analysis was carried out using the following criteria **[43]** :

- The drug speciality: EPREX® or another speciality ;
- Route of administration: subcutaneous (SC) or intravenous (IV);
- Type of packaging: pre-filled syringes or vials;
- Nature of stabilizing excipient: polysorbate 80 or human serum albumin.

At the end of this analysis, Boven et *al.* found that **[43]**:

- In the period from January 1'1989 to June 30, 2004, 217 cases of EMA were reported in CKD patients, with a notable incidence in 1998. In addition, only 183 patients were treated solely with EPREX® , while 23 received EPREX® with another speciality during their treatment, prior to the onset of PRCA.
- Of the 206 patients treated with EPREX® , 192 received it as SC injections, 9 received both SC and IV administration, while for the remaining 5 patients, the route of administration was not mentioned. It

should also be noted that no cases of EMA were reported when EPREX® was administered exclusively by IV.

- Of the 206 patients treated with EPREX® , 183 received their treatment in pre-filled syringes. Data for the remainder were unavailable.
- Of the 206 patients treated with EPREX® , 196 used a formulation containing polysorbate 80 as stabilizer. For the others, the stabilizer used was human serum albumin.

In the light of these observations, the authors concluded that EMA associated with EPREX® is a multifactorial pathology **[43]**. However, one of the factors contributing significantly to its onset was the release of organic substances from the primary packaging (seals on pre-filled syringes). These substances, whose release is promoted by the excipient polysorbate 80, appear to potentiate the drug's immunogenicity in CKD patients receiving SC therapy. Thus, the IV administration of EPREX® , the use of human serum albumin as a stabilizer and the application of a coating to the seals could prevent iatrogenic PRCA.

### 4.3. Interactions between drugs and medical devices

Medical devices encompass a wide range of products that perform specific functions such as **[45]** :

- Disease diagnosis ;
- Controlling disease progression;
- Treatment or alleviation of disease;
- Replacing an anatomical structure;
- Replacing a physiological function;
- Examination of samples from the human body (blood, tissue, etc.).

Unlike drugs, DMs act on the human body by mechanisms other than pharmacological, immunological or metabolic ones**[45]**

Thanks to innovative surgical techniques and early disease diagnosis and monitoring, the use of DMs has revolutionized the management of patients with acute or chronic illnesses **[46]**. Today, although they are ubiquitous in the care pathway, DMs are not without risk, and multiple adverse events have occurred since their first use, particularly CCIs. These items, which are made of different materials, can interact with drugs and biological products, notably blood and blood derivatives, exposing patients to dangerous situations. Similarly, procedures such as drug infusion, blood transfusion, parenteral nutrition, dialysis and respiratory assistance are the most commonly involved **[47]**

Medical devices containing PVC were the first to be described in CCI contexts. Because of its physico-chemical properties (flexibility, stability), availability and cost-effectiveness, this material is used in the manufacture of tubing **[47]**. Cases of drug sorption by PVC tubing, and the release of toxic substances from PVC (whose plasticizer is bis(2-ethylhexyl) phthalate (DEHP)), have been widely described, both in the neonatal population and in adults.

At present, PVC and DEHP in particular are less and less involved in CCIs, given their restricted use due to their CMR (carcinogenic, mutagenic, reprotoxic) properties **[45,46]**. They have thus been replaced by other materials more compatible with drugs and biological products.

### 4.3.1. Cases of reversible sorption of immunosuppressants by central venous catheters

The central venous catheter (CVC) is an invasive medical device designed to be inserted percutaneously into a large-caliber vein, such as the internal jugular vein, subclavian vein or femoral vein [48]. The CVC is indicated in a variety of situations, including :

- **The administration of veno-aggressive drugs** such as vasopressors, chemotherapy or hypertonic solutions, which require administration in large-caliber veins to avoid vessel damage;
- **Mass transfusion of blood** and blood products, in situations where rapid and efficient access is essential;
- **Parenteral nutrition** for patients unable to absorb nutrients through the digestive tract;
- **Cases of insufficient peripheral venous capital**, when peripheral access is contraindicated or difficult;
- **Monitoring hemodynamic parameters**, such as central venous pressure, to assess the patient's circulatory status;
- **Frequent blood sampling** facilitates analysis without the need for repeated peripheral venipuncture.

Inserting and maintaining a CVC exposes patients to a variety of risks, including catheter obstruction, thrombosis, catheter-related infection, gas embolism and device rupture [48]. These risks are well known to healthcare professionals, who are familiar with preventive measures and the protocols to be followed in the event of a complication. However, other CVC-related risks, in particular those associated with CHF, have also been identified. Among them, cases of **drug sorption by the catheter** have been reported.

This phenomenon, which results in adsorption of the drug by the walls of the catheter, has led not only to loss of the quantity of drug administered, but also to errors in the measurement of its plasma concentration, compromising the efficacy of treatment and the accuracy of therapeutic monitoring.

One study demonstrated that sorption of cyclosporine and tacrolimus by CVCs resulted in falsely elevated plasma concentrations of these drugs **[49]**. The latter, immunosuppressants of the calcineurin inhibitor class, are indicated primarily to prevent and treat organ and stem cell transplant rejection **[50]**. Their efficacy depends on rigorous maintenance of plasma concentrations within a narrow therapeutic range. Any variation in dosage, whether over- or underdosing, exposes patients to potentially serious, even fatal, risks. These include renal toxicity, hypertension, severe infections, graft rejection and graft-versus-host disease.

Hacker et *al* **[49]** undertook a study into the phenomenon of reversible sorption of ciclosporin and tacrolimus by central venous catheters (CVCs), motivated by the discovery of a marked difference between tacrolimus concentrations measured in blood samples taken via a CVC and by venipuncture. In this particular case, the catheter had been used to administer tacrolimus to the patient prior to blood sampling. The concentration measured in the CVC sample was 86 µg/L, while that obtained by venipuncture was just 2.9 µg/L.

As a first step, the research team carried out an *in vitro* study to analyze the sorption of cyclosporine and tacrolimus in CVCs **[49]**. They simulated the intravenous administration of these drugs through CVCs and reproduced the blood collection process from these devices. The study involved three types of CVC: polyurethane, silicone, and polyurethane incorporating an antimicrobial agent. The researchers infused ciclosporin and tacrolimus solutions through these CVCs for 6 hours for ciclosporin and 22 hours for tacrolimus, with initial concentrations of 2.5 g/L and 40 mg/L, respectively. At the end of each infusion, simulated blood samples were drawn by injecting fresh frozen plasma through the catheters. Then, each catheter was flushed with sodium chloride (NaCl) solution, and samples were taken after each flush to measure drug residues.

Meanwhile, Hacker et *al.* conducted a prospective *in vivo* study **[49]** of 15 hospitalized patients, aged 22 to 68, receiving ciclosporin or tacrolimus therapy following stem cell transplantation. Of these, twelve patients were on cyclosporine and three on tacrolimus. The drugs were administered daily by infusion via a CVC over a 22-hour period, followed by a 2-hour rinse of 50 mL NaCl solution. After each NaCl rinse, blood samples were taken to assess immunosuppressant concentrations. For each patient, two separate samples were taken: one directly from the CVC used to infuse the drug, and the other by venipuncture, in order to compare the concentrations obtained by the two sampling methods. In both parts of the study (*in vitro* and *in vivo*), ciclosporin and tacrolimus concentrations were measured in duplicate, using high-performance liquid chromatography-mass spectrometry.

In the *in vitro* study, fresh-frozen plasma samples collected after passage through CVCs used for ciclosporin or tacrolimus infusion revealed variable concentrations of these drugs (ranging from 260 to 17,000 µg/L for ciclosporin and 93 to 395 µg/L for tacrolimus) **[49]**. All types of catheter tested showed an ability to adsorb and then release these drugs into plasma, with a particularly marked phenomenon in silicone CVCs compared with polyurethane ones, whether conventional or fitted with an antimicrobial agent. Furthermore, despite successive rinses of the CVCs with NaCl, tacrolimus concentrations in the simulated samples decreased but remained detectable, even after the use of large volumes of NaCl (up to 24 L).

For the *in vivo* studies, the concentrations of cyclosporine and tacrolimus measured in blood samples obtained via CVCs and venipuncture are summarized **in Table XII**.

In patients 1 to 11, plasma ciclosporin concentrations measured in blood samples taken via CVCs were 6.7 to 22 times higher than those obtained by venipuncture **[49]**. For patients 12 and 13, treated with tacrolimus, plasma concentrations were respectively 150 and 116 times higher in samples taken via CVCs than those obtained by venipuncture. Finally, in patients 14 and 15, in whom treatment was either replaced by an oral route or suspended, plasma concentrations measured via CVCs remained 3 times higher than those obtained by venipuncture.

**TableXII : Plasma concentrations of ciclosporin and tacrolimus on samples taken through CVCs and by venipuncture, according to [49].**

| Patient | Drug administered | Drug concentration in sample (µg/L) | |
|---|---|---|---|
| | | Venipuncture | Through HVAC |
| Patient 1 | Ciclosporin | 235 | 2490 |
| Patient 2 | Ciclosporin | 96 | 2110 |
| Patient 3 | Ciclosporin | 249 | 4410 |
| Patient 4 | Ciclosporin | 144 | 2255 |
| Patient 5 | Ciclosporin | 172 | 1615 |
| Patient 6 | Ciclosporin | 138 | 1460 |
| Patient 7 | Ciclosporin | 192 | 1755 |
| Patient 8 | Ciclosporin | 248 | 1655 |
| Patient 9 | Ciclosporin | 199 | 1990 |

| Patient 10 | Ciclosporin | 198 | 1635 |
|---|---|---|---|
| Patient 11 | Ciclosporin | 229 | 1930 |
| Patient 12 | Tacrolimus | 5,1 | 767 |
| Patient 13 | Tacrolimus | 6,1 | 705 |
| Patient 14* | Ciclosporin | 296 | 895 |
| Patient 15 | Tacrolimus | 12,9 | 37 |

Patient 14*: ciclosporin infusion was stopped in this patient and replaced by oral administration. Blood samples were taken 3 days after initiation of oral treatment.
Patient 15*: this patient had received a single dose of tacrolimus, after which treatment was suspended due to high plasma concentrations. Blood samples from this patient were taken 3 days after treatment suspension.

The results of *in vitro* and *in vivo* studies are concordant and confirm the initial hypothesis that CVCs, whatever their material of construction, adsorb ciclosporin and tacrolimus **[49]**. This adsorption is reversible, meaning that the drugs are gradually released into the fluids passing through the catheters, even several days after treatment has been administered. In the case of blood samples taken to monitor plasma concentrations of these drugs, the adsorption/desorption phenomenon at catheter level leads to falsely elevated plasma concentration results. Faced with these artificially high concentrations of calcineurin inhibitors, doctors may have to reduce the doses administered, which presents a risk of drug underdosing. In the case of immunosuppressants, underdosing can lead to serious consequences, such as graft-versus-host disease or graft rejection, particularly in solid organ transplantation. These results underline the importance of taking into account the impact of drug sorption in CVCs to avoid dosing errors and ensure patient safety.

Hacker et *al* **[49]** recommended that venipuncture blood sampling should be preferred to avoid bias due to drug sorption in CVCs. Another alternative for monitoring cyclosporin plasma concentrations is to use a multi-lumen catheter. This type of catheter, with its multiple pathways, enables the simultaneous administration of several drugs, including incompatible ones, by delivering them via separate routes. In this context, the team recommended taking blood samples from a different route to that used for drug administration, to minimize the potential impact of sorption on plasma concentration results.

### 4.3.2. Antibiotic adsorption on the extracorporeal membrane oxygenation circuit

Extracorporeal membrane oxygenation (ECMO) is a life-support technique of last resort, used in intensive care units to treat patients suffering from severe respiratory or cardiac failure **[51]**. In such cases, ECMO is installed to temporarily replace failing organs and allow them to rest, with a view to recovering their functions at a later date.

Generally speaking, ECMO involves oxygenating blood outside the body. The process involves conveying venous blood rich in carbon dioxide ($CO_2$) to the ECMO circuit, passing the blood through a membrane that acts as a pulmonary alveolus, oxygenating the blood and removing $CO_2$, reheating the oxygenated blood and returning it to the patient **[51]**. These different stages are carried out by various accessories, including :

- The blood pump, which circulates the blood in the circuit and regulates its flow;
- Endovascular cannulas: inserted into large vessels to transfer blood from the body to the circuit (drainage cannula) and vice versa (return cannula);

- The oxygenation membrane or gas exchange membrane, which oxygenates the blood and eliminates $CO_2$ ;
- The heat exchanger, which warms oxygenated blood and brings its temperature down to that of the body;
- The tubing that circulates blood through the circuit's various compartments.

Thanks to ECMO, patients in critical situations have been saved. Nevertheless, the use of this technique exposes them to high infectious risks. Indeed, the mortality rate for infections associated with ECMO has reached 68% **[52]**. Consequently, this technique requires the use of heavy biotherapies. The most commonly used molecules include fluconazole and voriconazole as antifungal agents, and vancomycin as an antibiotic.

The success of anti-infective treatment depends on the choice of anti-infective agent and the selection of the appropriate dose **[53]**. The latter may be influenced by the patient's pathological factors and the DMs in contact with him/her. Indeed, it has been shown that ECMO can lead to changes in the pharmacokinetic parameters of drugs, increasing the volume of distribution and modifying clearance. In addition, drugs can be adsorbed by the circuit's various devices, reducing the dose administered to the patient. This adsorption is influenced by several factors: the nature of the components, the duration of the technique and the physicochemical properties of the drugs.

Aware of this phenomenon and its repercussions on patients on the one hand, and the scarcity of data and recommendations relating to it on the other, Raffaelli et *al.* conducted a study to elucidate the impact of ECMO on the quantities of voriconazole and vancomycin administered to patients **[54]**

The study, carried out *in vitro*, involved the installation of nine closed ECMO circuits for adults, children, infants and neonates. The circuits were connected to blood bags and maintained for 24 hours under physiological conditions.

First, blood was circulated through the circuits at variable flow rates and volumes, in the presence of heparin to prevent coagulation. Next, voriconazole and then vancomycin were injected in separate quantities. Blood samples were then taken to monitor changes in the levels of these anti-infectives ($T_0$, $T_{(2min)}$, $T_{(10min)}$, $T_{(30min)}$, $T_{(180min)}$, $T_{(360min)}$ and $T_{(24hours)}$ corresponding to the end of the experiment) **[54]**

After centrifugation, plasma supernatants from the various samples were collected in polypropylene vials sealed with polyethylene caps. Plasma concentrations of anti-infectives were measured by LC-MS **[54]**

A total of 72 samples (8 for each circuit) were analyzed.

In their final report, the authors mentioned that after 24 hours of circulation in the circuit, the average recovery percentages were 20% and 62% for voriconazole and vancomycin respectively **[54]**. In other words, between 38% and 80% of the product was retained (adsorbed) by the circuit. Unlike voriconazole, where the phenomenon was stable across different circuit categories, adsorption was circuit-dependent for vancomycin.

According to Raffaelli et *al.* this difference is mainly due to the physicochemical properties of the two molecules: voriconazole is highly lipophilic, while vancomycin is hydrophilic. This phenomenon exposes patients to sub-therapeutic concentrations, and consequently to therapeutic failure and microbial resistance. The authors therefore recommended pharmacological therapeutic monitoring when vancomycin or voriconazole therapy is initiated in patients on ECMO, in order to adjust dosage if necessary, and in the case of voriconazole, they suggested increasing the dose administered.

### 4.3.3. Bisphenol A release during dialysis

2,2-bis (4-hydroxyphenyl) propane, commonly known as Bisphenol A (BPA), is a ubiquitous organic compound found in a wide range of everyday consumer products **[55]**. BPA is mainly used in the manufacture of thermoplastics and thermosetting plastics, such as polycarbonate, polysulfone and epoxy resins. These materials are then used to produce food packaging (cans, bottles, etc.), medical devices, toys, electronics and many other everyday products.

However, it has been shown that BPA can migrate from materials containing it and accumulate in contact products such as foodstuffs **[55]**. When products contaminated with BPA are consumed, it accumulates in the body and can cause toxic effects. Research has shown that BPA has endocrine activity, which may be responsible for a variety of disorders, such as liver, respiratory and thyroid abnormalities, as well as cognitive and behavioral problems. It has also been associated with serious pathologies such as obesity, diabetes, certain cancers, as well as embryonic development abnormalities. More recently, studies have revealed that blood levels of BPA are correlated with an increased risk of developing chronic renal failure.

Competent authorities have taken action in response to the risks posed by BPA to human health **[55]**. This compound has been classified as an endocrine disruptor by the European Chemicals Agency, leading to worldwide restrictions on its use. For example, in the European Union:

- In 2011, a ban on the use of BPA in the manufacture of polycarbonate baby bottles was introduced;
- In 2013, this ban was extended to the manufacture of polycarbonate containers intended for the feeding of infants and children under 3 years of age;
- In 2023, the European Food Safety Authority (EFSA) significantly reduced the tolerable daily intake of BPA from 4 μg/kg/day to 0.2 ng/kg/day, a reduction by a factor of 20,000.

Nevertheless, the use of BPA in medical devices has not been restricted, despite recommendations to this effect **[55]**. In 2016, the European Scientific Committee on Emerging and Newly Identified Health Risks recommended the replacement of BPA by other substances in the manufacture of DM intended for infants, intensive care units and dialysis treatments. However, BPA is still present in these different categories of devices. Dialysis DMs, in particular, are causing concern in the scientific community, as patients suffering from chronic renal failure and receiving dialysis treatment are considered to be the most vulnerable to the toxic effects of BPA.

In a recent study, a group of researchers sought to confirm the overexposure of dialysis patients to endocrine disruptors, in particular BPA **[56]**. The team first compared BPA blood concentrations between three groups of participants:

- Group 1: 64 patients with end-stage renal disease on dialysis;
- Group 2: 36 non-dialyzed patients with end-stage renal disease;
- Group 3: 24 healthy volunteers.

The concentration of BPA in blood was measured using ultra-high performance liquid chromatography coupled with tandem mass spectrometry

**[56]**. The results showed that BPA was detected in blood samples from all patients in group 1 (dialysis patients), as well as in around 50% of participants in groups 2 (non-dialysis patients) and 3 (healthy volunteers). In addition, plasma BPA concentrations were significantly higher in blood samples from group 1 patients, with levels 22.5 times higher than in healthy volunteers and 1.4 times higher than in group 2 patients. On this basis, Cambien et *al.* concluded that CKD patients are more exposed to BPA than healthy subjects, and that, among these patients, those on dialysis have the highest exposure.

To assess the impact of dialysis on plasma BPA concentrations, Cambien et *al* **[56]** measured BPA levels before and after a dialysis session. The results showed that plasma BPA concentration did not change significantly, suggesting that dialysis does not effectively remove BPA from the blood. Several factors may explain this phenomenon:

- **The molecular weight of BPA**: As a low-molecular-weight molecule, some filtered BPA can be reabsorbed into the bloodstream during dialysis.
- **Binding of BPA to albumin**: As a portion of BPA is bound to albumin, it cannot pass through the dialyzer's filtration membrane.
- **The ubiquity of BPA**: BPA is present in various components of the dialyzer, such as filters, housings, dialysate and replacement fluid. Consequently, additional quantities of BPA can be introduced into the bloodstream during dialysis, compensating for any losses due to filtration.

Subsequently, Cambien et *al* **[56]** evaluated the impact of dialyzer construction materials on plasma BPA concentrations. They found that the presence of polysulfone in dialyzer filters led to an increase in these concentrations. Indeed, polysulfone is well known for its ability to release BPA, while materials such as cellulose and polynephron have lower release properties, thus reducing BPA exposure.

In conclusion, end-stage renal failure patients treated with hemodialysis are particularly vulnerable to exposure to endocrine disruptors, particularly BPA, compared to the general population. This overexposure results not only from the inability of their kidneys to effectively eliminate this substance, but also from the continuous introduction of BPA during dialysis sessions, due to the materials used in dialysis devices and the persistence of this molecule in their bloodstream.

## CONCLUSION

Container-content interactions are critical physico-chemical phenomena that occur in various fields, including pharmaceuticals. These interactions threaten the quality, efficacy, stability and safety of drugs, thereby compromising their therapeutic integrity.

In this thesis, we first analyzed the mechanisms of CCIs, showing that they manifest themselves through different types of substance transfer (sorption, release, permeation), each influenced by factors related to the container, contents and conditions of use. We then explored the regulatory requirements developed at international level to limit these interactions, highlighting the contributions of the European and American pharmacopoeias and directives aimed at framing and improving the assessment of pharmaceutical packaging. Finally, we studied concrete cases of CCI at each stage of the drug life cycle, showing that materials such as plastics and elastomers are the most conducive to these phenomena.

Despite significant progress in materials manufacturing and the implementation of early assessment strategies, CCIs remain a challenge for the pharmaceutical industry. However, preventive efforts have significantly reduced the frequency and impact of certain interactions, while increasingly powerful analytical techniques offer improved detection and understanding of CCIs.

The future of CCI research and practice is looking bright, thanks to technological advances such as the growing integration of predictive models based on artificial intelligence. These models make it possible to anticipate possible interactions between drugs and materials more accurately and rapidly, reducing the need to rely exclusively on conventional experimental protocols. As these predictive methods become more accurate, the sector could not only improve the safety and quality of pharmaceutical products, but also optimize container design and validation processes.

Ultimately, although CCIs are still a complex reality to manage, the development of new approaches to real-time simulation and analysis, combined with innovative materials, points to a future where harmful interactions could be almost entirely anticipated and controlled. The pharmaceutical sector is thus at the dawn of an era of more proactive CCI management, based on predictive technologies and strengthened collaboration between researchers, industry and regulatory authorities. These collective efforts will ensure better patient protection, while promoting responsible and effective innovation in pharmaceutical packaging.

# BIBLIOGRAPHICAL REFERENCES


1. Laschi A, Senhal N, Alarcon A, Barcelo B, Caire-Maurisier F, Delaire M, et al. Container-content interaction. II. Méthodologie. STP Pharma Pratiques. 2007;17:143-60.
2. Royce A, Sykes G. Losses of bacteriostats from injections in rubber-closed containers. J Pharm Pharmacol. 1957;9:814-22.
3. Moorhatch P, Chiou WL. Interactions between drugs and plastic intravenous fluid bags. I. Sorption studies on 17 drugs. Am J Hosp Pharm. 1974;31:72-8.
4. Cuadros-Rodríguez L, Lazúen-Muros M, Ruiz-Samblás C, Navas-Iglesias N. Leachables from plastic materials in contact with drugs. State of the art and review of current analytical approaches. Int J Pharm. 2020;583:119332.
5. Murdan S. Packaging and stability of pharmaceutical products. In: Aulton ME, Taylor KMG, editors. Pharmaceutics: The design and manufacture of medicines. 5th ed. London: Elsevier; 2018. p. 820-35.
6. Swift R, Schaut R, Flynn CR, Asselta R. Glass containers for parenteral products. In: Nema S, Ludwig JD, editors. Parenteral medications. 4th ed. New York: CRC Press; 2019. p. 425-47.
7. United States Pharmacopeia. General Chapter ⟨1660⟩: Evaluation of the Inner Surface Durability of Glass Containers. In: United States Pharmacopeia and National Formulary. Rockville: USP; 2024.
8. European Directorate for the Quality of Medicines and Healthcare. Containers. In: European Pharmacopoeia. 10th ed. Strasbourg: EDQM; 2019. p. 491-499.

9. Waxman L, De Grazio FL, Vilivalam VD. Plastic packaging for parenteral drug delivery. In: Nema S, Ludwig JD, editors. Parenteral medications. 4th ed. New York: CRC Press; 2019. p. 480-506.

10. United States Pharmacopeia. General Chapter 〈1381〉: Assessment of Elastomeric Component Used in Injectable Pharmaceutical Product Packaging/Delivery. In: United States Pharmacopeia and National Formulary. Rockville: USP; 2024.

11. Chennell P, Bernard L, Le Basle Y, Sautou V. Interactions between drugs and medical devices. In: Apnec, Aulagner G, Bedouch P, Sautou-Miranda V, directeurs. Clinical pharmacy and medical devices. Paris: Elsevier Health Sciences; 2023.p. 57-61.

12. United States Pharmacopeia. General Chapter 〈1664〉: Assessment of drug product leachables associated with pharmaceutical packaging/delivery systems. In: United States Pharmacopeia and National Formulary. Rockville: USP; 2024.

13. Tokhadzé N. Study of sorption phenomena between perfusion drugs and medical devices: empirical and fundamental approach by molecular simulation [Thesis]. Clermont-Ferrand: Université Clermont Auvergne; 2020.

14. Garde JA, Catalá R, Gavara R, Hernandez RJ. Characterizing the migration of antioxidants from polypropylene into fatty food simulants. Food Addit Contam. 2001;18(8):750-62.

**15.** United States Pharmacopeia. General Chapter ⟨1663⟩: Assessment of Extractables Associated with Pharmaceutical Packaging/Delivery Systems. In: United States Pharmacopeia and National Formulary. Rockville: USP; 2024.

**16.** Lau OW, Wong SK. Contamination in food from packaging material. J Chromatogr A. 2000;882(1):255-70.

**17.** Smith EJ, Paskiet DM, Tullo EJ. The Management of extractables and leachables in pharmaceutical products. In: Nema S, Ludwig JD, editors. Parenteral medications. 4th ed. New York: CRC Press; 2019. p. 536-70.

**18.** Feutry F. Étude des interactions physico-chimiques entre les préparations parentérales et un nouveau conditionnement primaire utilisable en unité de préparation centralisée, le flacon Crystal® [Thesis]. Lille: Université du Droit et de la Santé - Lille II; 2016.

**19.** Food and Drug Administration. Guidance for industry: container closure systems for packaging human drugs and biologics. Rockville: U.S. Department of Health and Human Services; 1999.

**20.** Jenke D. Extactables and leachables: characterization of drug products, packaging, manufacturing and delivery systems, and medical devices. Hoboken: Wiley; 2022.

**21.** Laschi A, Senhal N, Alarcon A, Barcelo B, Caire-Maurisier F, Delaire M, et al. Container-content interaction. I. Réglementation. STP Pharma Pratiques. 2007;17:131-41.

**22.** US Pharmacopeia. USP timeline [Online]. Rockville: US Pharmacopeia; 2024 [accessed September 23, 2024]. Available: https://www.usp.org/200-anniversary/usp-timeline.

**23.** United States Pharmacopeia. General Chapter ⟨659⟩: Packaging and Storage. In: United States Pharmacopeia and National Formulary. Rockville: USP; 2024.

**24.** United States Pharmacopeia. General Chapter ⟨1661⟩: Evaluation of Plastic Packaging Systems for Pharmaceutical Use and Their Materials of Construction. In: United States Pharmacopeia and National Formulary. Rockville: USP; 2024.

**25.** United States Pharmacopeia. General Chapter ⟨661.2⟩: Plastic Packaging Systems for Pharmaceutical Use. In: United States Pharmacopeia and National Formulary. Rockville: USP; 2024.

**26.** United States Pharmacopeia. General Chapter ⟨87⟩: Biological Reactivity Tests, *in vitro*. In: United States Pharmacopeia and National Formulary. Rockville: USP; 2024.

**27.** United States Pharmacopeia. General Chapter ⟨1664.1⟩: Orally Inhaled and Nasal Drug Products. In: United States Pharmacopeia and National Formulary. Rockville: USP; 2024.

**28.** United States Pharmacopeia. General Chapter ⟨381⟩: Elastomeric Components in Injectable Pharmaceutical Product Packaging/Delivery Systems. In: United States Pharmacopeia and National Formulary. Rockville: USP; 2024.

**29.** Convention on the Elaboration of a European Pharmacopoeia. Strasbourg : Council of Europe ; July 22 1964.

30. European Directorate for the Quality of Medicines and Healthcare. General requirements. In: European Pharmacopoeia. 10th ed. Strasbourg: EDQM; 2019. p. 3-11.
31. European Directorate for the Quality of Medicines and Healthcare. Materials used in the manufacture of containers. In: European Pharmacopoeia. 10th ed. Strasbourg: EDQM; 2019. p. 459-486.
32. European Directorate for the Quality of Medicines and Healthcare. Containers for human blood and blood components, and materials used in their manufacture; transfusion sets and materials used in their manufacture; syringes. In: Pharmacopée Européenne. 10th ed. Strasbourg: EDQM; 2019. p. 505-518.
33. European Commission. EudraLex - Volume 3 - Scientific guidelines for medicinal products for human use [Online]. Brussels: European Commission; [cited 2 Nov 2024]. Available:https://health.ec.europa.eu/medicinal-products/eudralex/eudralex-volume-3_en
34. European Medicines Agency. Guideline on plastic immediate packaging materials. London: EMA; 2005.
35. Hammond M, Marghitoiu L, Lee H, Perez L, Rogers G, Nashed-Samuel Y, et al. A cytotoxic leachable compound from single-use bioprocess equipment that causes poor cell growth performance. Biotechnol Prog. 2014;30(2):332-7.
36. Hammond M, Nunn H, Rogers G, Lee H, Marghitoiu AL, Perez L, et al. Identification of a leachable compound detrimental to cell growth in

single-use bioprocess containers. PDA J Pharm Sci Technol. 2013;67:123-34.

**37.**Sacha GA, Saffell-Clemmer W, Abram K, Akers MJ. Practical fundamentals of glass, rubber, and plastic sterile packaging systems. Pharm Dev Technol. 2010;15:6-34.

**38.**Thakare V, Mayr B, Artenjak A, Nianios D, Sest M, Müller M, et al. Investigation of drug product and container-closure interactions: A case study of diluent containing prefilled syringe. Eur J Pharm Biopharm. 2019;140:67-77.

**39.**Marasini S, Craig JP, Dean SJ, Leanse LG. Managing Corneal Infections: Out with the old, in with the new? Antibiotics. 2023;12(8):1334.

**40.**Gollapalli R, Singh G, Blinder A, Brittin J, Sengupta A, Mondal B, et al. Identification of an adduct impurity of an active pharmaceutical ingredient and a leachable in an ophthalmic drug product using LC-QTOF. J Pharma Sci. 2019;108:3187-93.

**41.**Pan C, Liu F, Motto M. Identification of pharmaceutical impurities in formulated dosage forms. J Pharma Sci. 2011;100:1228-59.

**42.**Lobbes H. PRCA: diagnosis, classification, treatment. Rev Med Interne. 2023;44:19-26.

**43.**Boven K, Stryker S, Knight J, Thomas A, Regenmortel M, Kemeny DM, et al. The increased incidence of pure red cell aplasia with an EPREX® formulation in uncoated rubber stopper syringes. Kidney Int. 2005;67:2346-53.

**44.**Sharma B, Bader F, Templeman T, Lisi P, Ryan M, Heavner G. Technical investigation into the cause of the increased incidence of anti-body-mediated pure red cell aplasia associated with EPREX®. Eur J Hosp Pharm. 2004;5:86-91.

**45.**Regulation of the European Parliament and of the Council of 5 April 2017. on medical devices. Official Journal of the European Union. 2017; L 117: 1-175.

**46.**Bedouch P, Aulagner G, Sautou V. Clinical pharmacy in the field of medical devices: Definition and issues. In: Aulagner G, Bedouch P, Sautou-Miranda V, directeurs. Clinical pharmacy and medical devices. Paris: Elsevier Health Sciences; 2023.p. 3-8.

**47.**Testai E, Hartemann P, Rastogi SC, Bernauer U, Piersma A, De Jong W, et al. The safety of medical devices containing DEHP plasticized PVC or other plasticizers on neonates and other groups possibly at risk (2015 update). Regul Toxicol Pharmacol. 2016;76:209-210.

**48.**Haubertin C, Poiroux L, Kouatchet A. The central venous catheter in intensive care. In: Decormeille G, Poiroux L, Dauvergne J, Constan A, Blanchard PY, Valera S, directeurs. L'infirmier(e) en service de réanimation. Paris: Elsevier; 2022.p. 179-82.

**49.**Hacker C, Verbeek M, Schneider H, Steimer W. Falsely elevated cyclosporin and tacrolimus concentrations over prolonged periods of time due to reversible adsorption to central venous catheters. Clin Chim Acta. 2014;433:62-8.

**50.**Parlakpinar H, Gunata M. Transplantation and immunosuppression: a review of novel transplant-related immunosuppressant drugs. Immuno pharmacol Immuno toxicol. 2021;43:651-65.

**51.**Wrisinger WC, Thompson SL. Basics of extracorporeal membrane Oxygenation. Surg Clin North Am. 2022;102:23-35.

**52.** Peña-López Y, Machado MC, Rello J. Infection in ECMO patients: Changes in epidemiology, diagnosis and prevention. Anaesth Crit Care Pain Med. 2024;43:101319.

**53.** Zhang Y, Zeng Z, Zhang Q, Ou Q, Chen Z. Effect of extracorporal membrane oxygenation on pharmacokinetics of antimicrobial Drugs: recent progress and recommendations. J South Med Univ. 2021;41:793-800.

**54.** Raffaeli G, Gavallaro G, Allegaert K, et al. Sequestration of voriconazole and vancomycin into contemporary extracorporeal membrane oxygenation circuits: An *in vitro* Study. Front Pediatr. 2020;8:468.

**55.** González-Parra E, Moreno-Gómez-Toledano R, Mas-Fontao S, Bosch R. Bisphenol A in renal insufficiency: how long will it be used? Is it time to avoidit? Nefrología (English Edition). 2024;44(3):313-16.

**56.** Cambien G, Dupuis A, Belmouaz M, Bauwens M, Bacle A, Ragot S, et al. Bisphenol A and chlorinated derivatives of bisphenol A assessment in end stage renal disease patients: Impact of dialysis therapy. Ecotoxicol Environ Saf. 2024;270:115880.

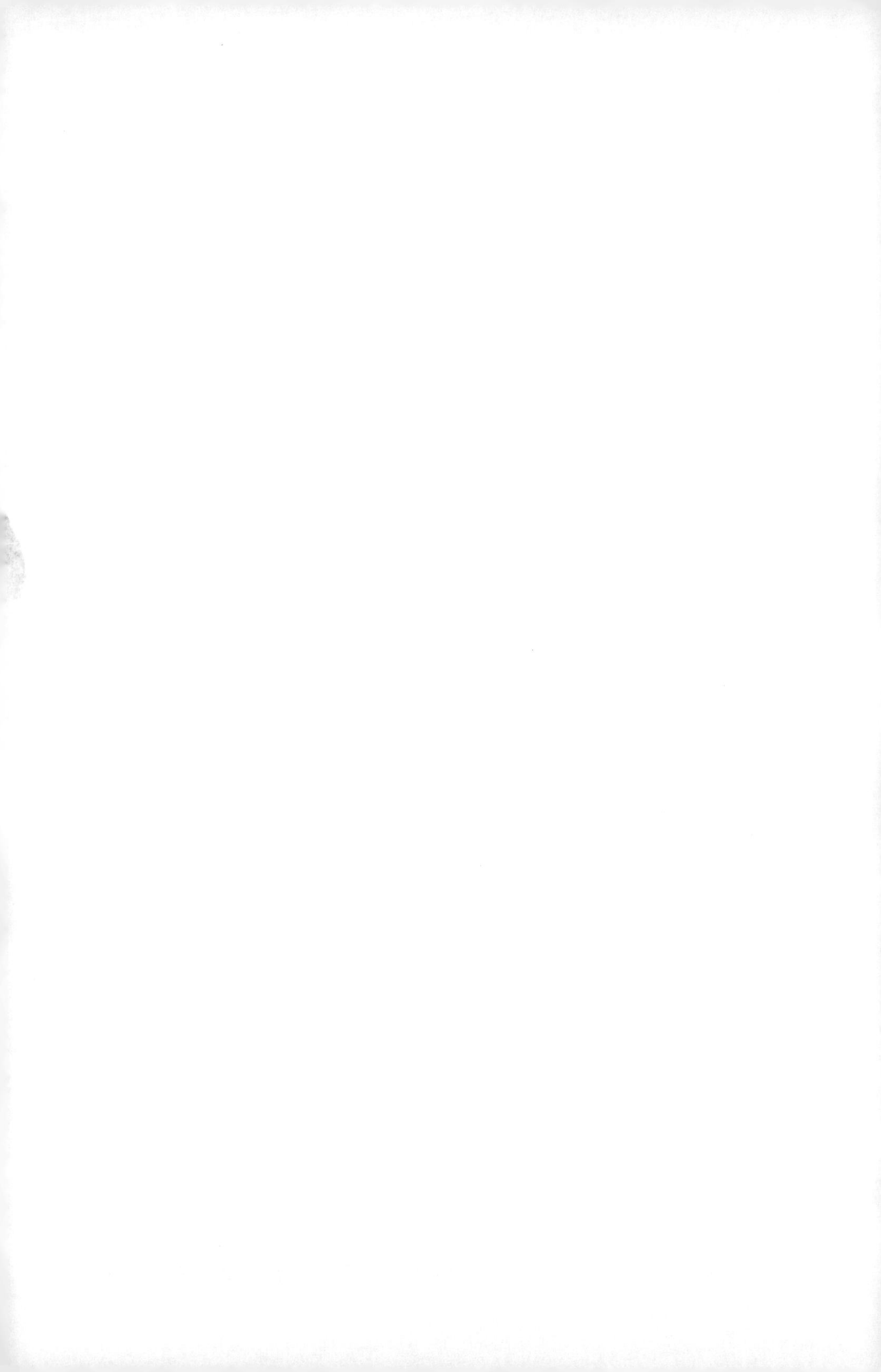

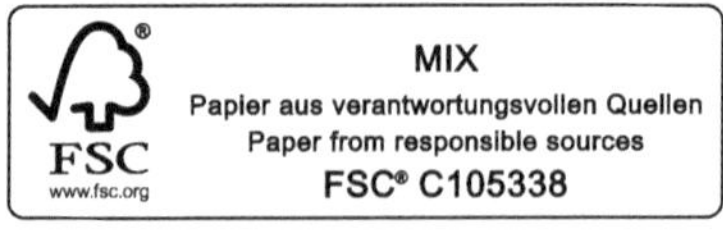


Printed by Books on Demand GmbH, Norderstedt / Germany